Nursing Adults with Long Term Conditions

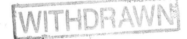

Transforming Nursing Practice series

Transforming Nursing Practice is the first series of books designed to help students meet the requirements of the NMC Standards and Essential Skills Clusters for degree programmes. Each book addresses a core topic, and together they cover the generic knowledge required for all fields of practice. Accessible and challenging, *Transforming Nursing Practice* helps nursing students prepare for the demands of future healthcare delivery.

Core knowledge titles:

Personal and professional learning skills titles:

To order, contact our distributor: BEBC Distribution, Albion Close, Parkstone, Poole, BH12 3LL. Telephone: 0845 230 9000, email: learningmatters@bebc.co.uk. You can also find more information on each of these titles and our other learning resources at www.learningmatters.co.uk. Many of these titles are also available in various e-book formats, please visit our website for more information.

Nursing Adults with Long Term Conditions

Jane Nicol

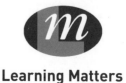

Learning Matters

First published in 2011 by Learning Matters Ltd

British Library Cataloguing in Publication Data
A CIP record for this book is available from the British Library

ISBN: 978 0 85725 441 2

This book is also available in the following ebook formats:

Adobe ebook ISBN: 978 0 857254436
ePub ebook ISBN: 978 0 857254429
Kindle ISBN: 978 0 857254443

Cover and text design by Toucan Design
Project management and typesetting by 4word Ltd, Page & Print Production
Printed and bound in Great Britain by Short Run Press Ltd, Exeter, Devon

Learning Matters Ltd
20 Cathedral Yard
Exeter EX1 1HB
Tel: 01392 215560
E-mail: info@learningmatters.co.uk
www.learningmatters.co.uk

FSC
www.fsc.org
MIX
Paper from
responsible sources
FSC® C014540

Contents

About the author

Jane Nicol is a registered nurse and Senior Lecturer at the University of Worcester. During her career she has worked across a range of clinical settings, enabling her to develop a broad knowledge and skill base. She currently teaches on the pre-registration nursing programme at the University of Worcester, focusing on the care and management of people living with a long term condition and people receiving palliative care. Her particular areas of interest are interpersonal and intrapersonal skills, and the importance of these in allowing nurses to develop positive relationships with the people for whom they care.

Acknowledgements

The publishers and author would like to thank the following for their very helpful feedback during the writing of this book:

Maggie Roberts, Health Lecturer and Pathway Leader for Primary Care, and Chair of the Community Practice Learning Team, at the University of Nottingham;

Paul Macreth, Senior Lecturer and Course Leader for District Nursing, at Leeds Metropolitan University.

They would also like to thank Pilgrim Projects Ltd and the Patient Voices website (**www. patientvoices.org.uk**) for Bill's story and the accompanying word cloud (Figure 2.1) in the case study on page 29. The word cloud was created at **www.wordle.net.**

Introduction

Those living with a long term condition (LTC) are often experts in their own condition, living with and managing it on a day-to-day basis. Therefore, nurses caring for and working with people living with an LTC have to possess the knowledge, skills and attributes that will foster partnership working, encourage self-management and support those whose condition requires more active care and management. While the chapters in this book are presented sequentially, it is recognised that aspects of the care and management of individuals living with an LTC, such as health promotion, feature throughout, from diagnosis through to palliative care.

Who is this book for?

This book is primarily for students of adult nursing, whether on a diploma or degree pathway. However, it is also aimed at supporting the development of knowledge for use in all fields of practice. Therefore, there may well be value for those who are studying in the field of child, mental health and learning disability and those on continuing professional development modules. It may also be of interest to experienced nurses who have mentoring roles. The Nursing and Midwifery Council's *Standards for Pre-registration Nursing Education* (NMC, 2010) are a foundation for what follows. However, the content is not narrowly defined by them.

A note on terminology

Given that the underlying premise of the care and management of long term conditions is based on self-care and self-management, the term 'person/individual' has been used, but when the context demands, the term 'patient' has been used.

Standards for Pre-registration Nursing Education and Essential Skills Clusters

These Standards (NMC, 2010) are used by those planning pre-registration nursing education courses. At the beginning of each chapter there is a guide to the most relevant domains and competencies described in the standards. However, this may not be exhaustive and readers should consult the full standards to support their own learning. The four domains, with their respective generic standards for competence, are as follows.

1. Domain 1: Professional values
   - All nurses must act first and foremost to care for and safeguard the public. They must practise autonomously and be responsible and accountable for safe, compassionate,

person-centred, evidence-based nursing care that respects and maintains dignity and human rights. They must show professionalism and integrity and work within recognised professional, ethical and legal frameworks. They must work in partnership with other health and social care professionals and agencies, service users, their carers and families in all settings, including the community, ensuring that decisions about care are shared.

2. Domain 2: Communication and interpersonal skills
   - All nurses must use excellent communication and interpersonal skills. Their communications must always be safe, effective, compassionate and respectful. They must communicate effectively using a wide range of strategies and interventions including the effective use of communication technologies. Where people have a disability, nurses must be able to work with service users and others to obtain the information they need to make reasonable adjustments that promote optimum health and enable equal access to services.

3. Domain 3: Nursing practice and decision-making
   - All nurses must practise autonomously, compassionately, skilfully and safely, and must maintain dignity and promote health and wellbeing. They must assess and meet the full range of essential physical and mental health needs of people of all ages who come into their care. Where necessary they must be able to provide safe and effective immediate care to all people prior to accessing or referring to specialist services irrespective of their field of practice. All nurses must be able to meet more complex and coexisting needs for people in their own nursing field of practice, in any setting including hospital, community and at home. All practice should be informed by the best available evidence and comply with local and national guidelines. Decision-making must be shared with service users, carers and families and informed by critical analysis of a full range of possible interventions, including the use of up-to-date technology. All nurses must also understand how behaviour, culture, socioeconomic and other factors, in the care environment and its location, can affect health, illness, health outcomes and public health priorities and take into account planning and delivering care.

4. Domain: Leadership, management and team working
   - All nurses must be professionally accountable and use clinical governance processes to maintain and improve nursing practice and standards of healthcare. They must be able to respond autonomously and confidently to planned and uncertain situations, managing themselves and others effectively. They must create and maximise opportunities to improve service. They must also demonstrate the potential to develop further management and leadership skills during their period of preceptorship and beyond.

The NMC states that the essential skills clusters (ESCs) must be part of all pre-registration nursing courses. How this is done is up to those who are planning how the course will be delivered. There are five skills clusters in total:

- care, compassion and communication;
- organisational aspects of care;
- infection prevention and control;
- nutrition and fluid management;
- medicines management.

These ESCs are designed to support the achievement of the competencies listed under each of the four domains. Some chapters in this book are particularly relevant to certain clusters, and this will be highlighted as appropriate.

Book structure

In Chapter 1, 'Long term conditions across the lifespan', the impact of LTCs across the lifespan is explored. What LTCs are, how care is delivered in the UK and the impact LTCs have on the individual, both physically and psychologically, are examined. To support the delivery of care in LTCs across the lifespan consideration will be given to the transition of care from child to adult services.

Chapter 2, 'The therapeutic relationship in long term conditions', emphasises the importance of developing and maintaining an effective therapeutic relationship with both the person living with an LTC and their carer. To do this the term emotional intelligence is outlined and its relevance to the therapeutic relationship in LTCs explained. The importance of effective communication is explored with some useful communication strategies being outlined and related to LTCs.

Chapter 3, 'Health promotion in long term conditions', uses an exploration of determinants of health and public health to set the context of health promotion in LTCs. This approach demonstrates the multifactorial nature of health and health promotion. The importance of health promotion in LTCs will be explained and applied to practice; health promotion models are outlined and their relevance to LTCs discussed. Strategies for health promotion such as motivational interviewing will be examined and related to people living with an LTC.

Chapter 4 focuses on the importance of promoting self-management and empowerment in long term conditions, for people living with an LTC. It emphasises the importance of empowerment and looks at how this can be promoted for people living with an LTC. By examining the skills and knowledge necessary to become successful self-managers, and by applying them to clinical scenarios, autonomy and empowerment of people living with LTCs will be increased.

Chapter 5 looks at quality of life and symptom management in long term conditions, highlighting the areas of a person's life that influence and affect their quality of life. Effective symptom management, as a strategy to improve and maintain quality of life, is discussed using the nursing process as a framework to support care. Emphasis is placed on effective medicines management, nutritional support and pain management. The nursing process is related to a clinical scenario and used as a framework for effective symptom management.

In Chapter 6, 'Managing complex care in long term conditions', the focus is on case management. The roles and responsibilities of case managers are reflected on, explored and related to case scenarios. Strategies to support complex care, such as care pathways and effective discharge planning, emphasise the need for collaborative working in the care and management of people living with an LTC.

Chapter 7 discusses the transition from active to palliative care in long term conditions, and emphasises the importance of effective communication when breaking 'bad news'. Relevant policy, legislation and strategies aimed at raising awareness of palliative care will be discussed.

Assessment frameworks are related to clinical scenarios to demonstrate the holistic nature of palliative care.

Learning features

This book provides a variety of learning features, including activities, research summaries, further reading and useful websites, to enable you to participate in, and guide, your own learning. A glossary of terms is included, explaining terms and ideas covered in the chapters. Glossary terms are in bold text the first time they appear. There are also four case studies which you will follow throughout the book. These have been collated into one useful document which is available on the Learning Matters website at **www.learningmatters.co.uk/nursing**. Click on the book in the full list of Nursing and Midwifery titles to access the link to this resource.

Chapter 1
Long term conditions across the lifespan

```
      NMC Standards for Pre-registration Nursing Education
```

This chapter will address the following competencies:

Domain 1: Professional values

3. All nurses must support and promote the health, wellbeing, rights and dignity of
    people, groups, communities and populations. These include people whose lives are
    affected by ill health, disability, ageing, death and dying. Nurses must understand how
    these activities affect public health.

Domain 3: Nursing practice and decision-making

2. All nurses must possess a broad knowledge of the structure and functions of the
    human body, and other relevant knowledge from the life, behavioural and social
    sciences as applied to health, ill health, disability, ageing and death. They must
    have an in-depth knowledge of common physical and mental health problems and
    treatments in their own field of practice, including co-morbidity and physiological
    and psychological vulnerability.

```
      NMC Essential Skills Clusters
```

This chapter will address the following ESCs:

Cluster: Organisational aspects of care

9. People can trust the newly registered graduate nurse to treat them as partners and
    work with them to make a holistic and systematic assessment of their needs; to
    develop a personalised plan that is based on mutual understanding and respect for
    their individual situation promoting health and wellbeing, minimising risk of harm
    and promoting safety at all times.

By the second progression point:

3. Understands the concept of public health and the benefits of healthy lifestyles
    and the potential risks involved with various lifestyles and behaviours, for example,
    substance misuse, smoking, obesity.

5. Contributes to care based on an understanding of how the different stages of an
    illness or disability can impact on people and carers.

Chapter aims

After reading this chapter you will be able to:

- describe the difference between a long term condition (LTC) and an acute condition;
- discuss the incidence of long term conditions and their impact on healthcare provision;
- understand how the care and management of people living with a long term condition are organised;
- reflect on the physical and psychological impacts of living with an LTC;
- recognise the importance of appropriate care during the transition from child to adult services.

Introduction

The life you had imagined for your child changes, uncertainty creeps in – are they going to be able to do all that you had hoped? It is on your mind all the time, you worry for their future.

(Quote from a parent of a child, aged eight, diagnosed with Type 1 diabetes)

I half expected it really, well with my previous lifestyle it kind of goes with the territory. Still nothing prepares you for the shock of hearing it, yes I know treatments are more effective now, but you still worry about the future.

(Young male (25) diagnosed with human immunodeficiency virus (HIV))

It was like losing Dad bit by bit, it was hard watching the effect that had on Mum. At the end though, it wasn't Dad anymore – he wasn't there, we had all said goodbye to him a long time ago.

(Daughter whose father was diagnosed with Alzheimer's at 60)

The diagnosis of a long term condition (LTC) can occur at different stages across the lifespan, resulting in different implications for the person and their future and also for those caring for them. For a child and their family a diagnosis of Type 1 diabetes will mean a lifetime of adjustment and management of their condition. For the person diagnosed with HIV it may mean living with the stigma of their diagnosis and the implications of this for their future. For a person diagnosed with dementia the realisation of the cognitive deterioration that is to come and how to manage that may be the focus of their needs. Not only will their immediate concerns be different, the impact that their condition has on their day-to-day life will vary across the person's life, resulting in a variety of health needs, with the impact being felt physically, socially and psychologically. In order for you to effectively support people living with an LTC, their family and carers it is important to have an understanding of what LTCs are, their incidence across the lifespan and the frameworks used to guide their care and management. In order to do this the chapter will develop your knowledge and understanding about LTCs, including transition of care from child to adult services and the importance of recognising the physical and psychological impact of living with an LTC.

The Department of Health (DH) defines an LTC as: *A long term condition is one that cannot be cured but can be managed through medication and/or therapy* (www.dh.gov.uk/en/Healthcare/ Longtermconditions/index.htm).

Using the above quote as a starting point take some time to answer these questions.

- How many LTCs can you list?
- How do acute and long term conditions differ in relation to diagnosis, treatment, prognosis and outcome?

A brief outline answer is given at the end of the chapter.

Activity 1.1 has drawn your attention to the complex nature of LTCs, their varying signs and symptoms, care and management and prognosis. Over time the symptoms of the condition become worse and there is a gradual or sometimes sudden deterioration in the health and wellbeing of the person living with the condition. The incidence of LTCs is rising, not only in the UK but throughout the world.

The rising incidence and impact of LTCs in the UK

When the National Health Service was founded in 1948, life expectancy for a boy born in that year was 66 years and for a girl 71 years (DH, 2000). Online statistics available from the United Nations Statistics Division now place life expectancy in the UK for men at 78 years and for women at 82 years. Information from the Office for National Statistics (ONS) indicates that the population of the UK is ageing, with an increase in the percentage of the population over the age of 65 (ONS, 2010). This development has resulted in an increase in the incidence and prevalence of LTCs, which is compounded by the rise in conditions such as Type 2 diabetes, coronary heart disease, chronic liver disease, which are exacerbated by lifestyle choices (DH, 2008a). The DH estimates that, due to ageing alone, the numbers of people living with an LTC will double every decade. Presently there are 17.5 million adults living with an LTC in the UK (DH, 2005) and it is estimated that 15% of children under the age of five and 20% of children between the ages of five and 15 are living with an LTC (Drennan and Goodman, 2007). These figures include 10 million adults who are living with a neurological LTC, as well as one in six adults (and one in ten children) who are living with a mental health LTC (DH, 2000).

LTCs do not occur in isolation: 70% of people over the age of 65 who are affected by an LTC are living with more than one, and 25% of people living with an LTC have three or more. People living with an LTC are known to be intensive users of health and social care services. While there may be some regional variation between the countries in the UK, approximately 30% of the population say they are living with an LTC. This 30% of the population account for 52% of all GP appointments, 65% of all out-patient appointments and 72% of all in-patient bed days (DH, 2008a).

Activity 1.2 *Reflection*

Ali was diagnosed with chronic kidney disease at the age of 30, in association with uncontrolled hypertension. Early in his disease Ali was symptom-free and he was prescribed medication for his hypertension. Despite the efforts of the healthcare team and being offered smoking cessation support he continued to smoke. Despite monitoring of his blood pressure Ali's symptoms increased and when he was 40 he began to experience weight loss, muscle cramps and nausea. His **estimated glomerular filtration rate (eGFR)** was 17 and he was placed on the transplant list. While waiting for his transplant Ali had **continuous ambulatory peritoneal dialysis (CAPD)**, which he was able to have at home.

Following his transplant, at the age of 42, Ali's health improved and his condition remained stable for ten years. Ali was offered further support regarding smoking cessation but continued to smoke. Ali was now married and father to three young children.

Unfortunately Ali's transplant began to fail and by the time he was 53 he was having hospital haemodialysis. Eventually, through perseverance and with the ongoing support of his family the resources were available for him to have this at home. It was during this period of dialysis that Ali eventually stopped smoking, following encouragement from his family and healthcare team. At the age of 60 Ali was offered another transplant which he accepted; this was not as successful as his first due to his ongoing hypertension.

At the age of 66, six years later after ongoing problems, Ali's second kidney transplant failed. He decided not to go back onto dialysis, and as his health deteriorated Ali was cared for at home by his wife and family. At this time both Ali and his family were aware that his condition was terminal, with the aim of his care being to maintain his comfort and dignity.

Using the above case scenario answer the following questions.

- Over the course of his disease progression what health and social care services would Ali and his family access?
- What impact will Ali's LTC have on his family?

A brief outline answer is given at the end of the chapter.

Activity 1.2 emphasises the impact caring and managing LTCs has not only for health and social care services but for the family of the person living with the condition. Over the course of their life a person living with an LTC will have contact with many health and social care professionals. Their care may be delivered in a **primary**, **secondary** setting or **tertiary** care setting. However, this case scenario demonstrates that the majority of care is delivered in primary care by members of the primary healthcare team. To minimise the impact an LTC has on both health and social care services it is important to recognise the role that the person living with the LTC, and their family and carers, has in their care and management.

Policy review

The UK has recognised that effective care and management of LTCs are essential if the impact of these conditions is to be reduced and the quality of life for people living with an LTC is to be improved. Each country within the UK has published policy documents relating to the care and management of LTCs.

- England: *National Service Framework for Long Term Conditions* (DH, 2005a) and *Supporting People with Long Term Conditions: An NHS and Social Care Model to support local innovation and integration* (DH, 2005b).
- Northern Ireland: *Caring for People Beyond Tomorrow: A Strategic Framework for the Development of Primary Health and Social Care for Individuals, Families and Communities in Northern Ireland* (Department of Health, Social Services and Public Safety (DHSSPS), 2005) and *Response to Proposals for Health and Social Care Reform in Northern Ireland* (Long Term Conditions Alliance Northern Ireland (LTCANI), 2008).
- Scotland: *Long Term Conditions Collaborative: High Impact Changes* (The Scottish Government Health Delivery Directorate Improvement Support Team, 2009).
- Wales: *Designed to Improve Health and Management of Chronic Conditions in Wales: An integrated model and framework* (Department of Health and Social Services (DHSS), 2007).

All these documents outline the care and management people living with an LTC can expect, with most of this care and management taking place in primary care. This includes managing acute exacerbations, e.g. in chronic obstructive pulmonary disease (COPD). There is a clear emphasis placed on the importance of working with the person to provide patient-centred care, promote empowerment, self-care and management. As the LTC progresses, professionals are expected to deliver effective care and case management and preparation for palliative care requirements.

Another key policy driver in the care and management of LTCs is the Quality and Outcome Framework (QOF): this is part of the General Medical Services contract for general practice (GP) that was implemented in 2004. This points-based system rewards general practices for excellence in the following domains: clinical care, organisation, patient experience and additional services. Within the QOF the clinical care focuses on the successful management of the most common LTCs through the use of specific indicators (see Table 1.1).

Conditions listed on the QOF (listed alphabetically)	Examples of QOF indicators (listed alphabetically)
• Asthma • Atrial fibrillation • Cancer • Chronic kidney disease (CKD) • Chronic obstructive pulmonary disease • Coronary heart disease	• Achieving target blood pressure, e.g. maintaining a blood pressure of 150/90 for people with hypertension • Achieving target cholesterol level • Confirming diagnosis with objective measures, e.g. echocardiogram confirming heart failure

continued overleaf...

continued...

• Dementia	• Conditions-specific reviews, e.g. retinal screening for people with diabetes
• Depression	
• Diabetes mellitus	• Influenza immunization, e.g. for those with COPD
• Epilepsy	
• Heart failure	• Maintaining an accurate register of each condition – applicable to all LTCs
• Hypertension	
• Hypothyroid	• Measuring blood pressure
• Learning disability	• Measuring cholesterol
• Mental health	• Offering smoking cessation advice
• Obesity	• Other condition-specific outcomes, e.g. lifestyle advice for people with cardiovascular disease
• Palliative care	
• Smoking	
• Stroke and transient ischaemic attack (TIA)	• Recording person's smoking status
	• Specific therapy, e.g. lithium therapy for psychotic disorders
	• Taking condition-specific blood tests, e.g. thyroid function tests for those with hypothyroid

Table 1.1: Quality Outcome Framework LTCs and examples of performance indicators (NHS Employers, 2009)

To support these generic policy documents other conditions-specific literature is available. In England and Wales other condition-specific National Service Frameworks have been published. In England and Scotland both the National Institute for Health and Clinical Excellence (NICE) and the Scottish Intercollegiate Guidelines Network (SIGN) publish clinical guidelines outlining best practice on a number of LTCs. While these documents describe what care and management people living with an LTC can expect, they do not describe how services may be set up and the care delivered. To do this there are many models of service delivery that can be used.

A model of care to support people living with an LTC

Within the UK there are several theoretical frameworks that can be used to organise services and care in the management of LTCs (DH, 2005b, 2008b; DHSS, 2007; NHS Scotland, 2007). These frameworks focus on increasing the level of control and input a person living with an LTC has in relation to how services are delivered and in managing their condition. Both the DH and the DHSS reflect the Kaiser Permanente service delivery model in their models of management (DH, 2005b; DHSS, 2007) (see Figure 1.1). The Kaiser Permanente approach, which is also evident in the model of care delivery in Scotland and Northern Ireland, is underpinned by promoting health within the population as a whole, e.g. smoking cessation and healthy eating. For people with an LTC the approach includes self-care/support, disease/care management and case management.

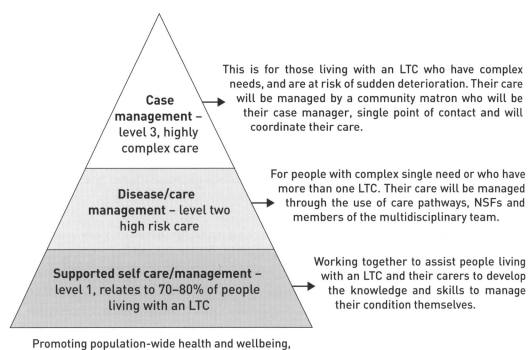

Figure 1.1: The NHS and Social Care long term conditions model
(Source: The pyramid structure is taken from DH, 2005b)

Examples of strategies that can be used in each of the areas of the triangle in Figure 1.1 include, for supported self-care/management, action planning, health promotion and assistive technology. For disease/care management strategies include personalised care planning, further support to enable self-management and access to specialist healthcare teams. In case management some of the strategies available include integrated assessment and care planning and risk assessment.

Activity 1.3   *Decision-making*

Read over the following case scenarios and decide which level of care on the Kaiser Permanente triangle best suits their current needs.

Angela (see website: www.learningmatters.co.uk/nursing for full case study)
Angela is 28 and was diagnosed with relapsing remitting multiple sclerosis (RRMS) following the birth of her son, Charlie, six months ago. She initially put her tiredness and aches and pains down to being a 'new mum'; however, she was persuaded by her husband, James, to see her GP. Following a series of investigations she was diagnosed with multiple sclerosis. Angela is still on maternity leave from her job as a librarian; she plans to return to work part time when Charlie is ten months old. She is finding caring for Charlie

continued overleaf...

continued...

tiring. James is helping out at home as much as he can as well as working as a computer software engineer for a local defence organisation.

Andrew (see website: www.learningmatters.co.uk/nursing for full case study)

Andrew is 75 years old, whose wife (Elizabeth) died ten years ago. He lives alone in a one-bedroomed flat in a sheltered housing complex. Andrew was diagnosed with COPD when he was 52 years old. He was a heavy smoker during his younger years, then he stopped for a while when he was 60 but started again after Elizabeth's death. Despite the efforts of his district nurse Andrew is still smoking. This has increased his dyspnoea and has resulted in a hospital admission due to recurring chest infections.

Frazer (see website: www.learningmatters.co.uk/nursing for full case study)

Frazer is 42 years old. He has Type 1 diabetes, which was diagnosed when he was eight years old. He lives with his long-term partner Claire and their daughter, Fiona, aged six. Frazer currently works part time as an office administrator and Claire works full time as a primary school teacher, Frazer works part time partly due to complications of his diabetes, mainly diabetic **polyneuropathy**, and partly to help out with childcare for Fiona. He is currently receiving treatment for an ulcer on his left foot that is slow to heal.

A brief outline answer is given at the end of the chapter

During the course of their disease progression people living with an LTC will move from one part of the triangle to another. As you can see from Activity 1.3, Andrew is currently in the disease/care management section. However, should his chest infections continue, and his health deteriorate, it may be that he progresses to the case management section of the triangle. A person living with an LTC can also move up and down the triangle. For example, following a relapse of her RRMS Angela may access specific disease or care management; then, once she has recovered from this she would return to supported self-care/management. This model of service delivery can be applied to any person living with any LTC. In line with this generic approach the DH has published information on generic models of care that can then be applied to any LTC. These include the following.

- *Generic choice model for long term conditions* (DH, 2007). With a focus on care planning, this model emphasises choice and control for a person living with an LTC. The following areas are seen as crucial to how a person living with an LTC is enabled to self-manage: what matters to the person and their carer, access to expert support and information and ensuring that any decisions made are done in partnership with the person.
- *Supporting People with Long Term Conditions: An NHS and Social Care Model to support local innovation and integration* (DH, 2005b). Using Kaiser Permanente as a framework (see Figure 1.1), this model promotes empowerment of the person living with an LTC through a supportive health care infrastructure, e.g. resources and delivery system, e.g. supporting self-care. The role that the primary health care team have in the care and management of people living with an LTC is emphasised within this model.

These models not only outline how services are to be delivered, they outline the roles and responsibilities that you and the person living with an LTC have in the care and management of their condition.

The impact of living with an LTC

As the quotations at the start of this chapter indicate, a diagnosis of an LTC can have a negative impact on the person and their family. Such a diagnosis is generally seen as being 'bad news', that is to say, news that implies the loss of something. The loss can relate to physical ability, loss of mobility due to motor neurone disease, something/someone that an individual values, altered body image (e.g. following mastectomy), which affects the way in which a person sees themselves, or loss of position in the family. The diagnosis of an LTC is usually given by a member of the medical profession. However, as a member of the healthcare team involved in that person's care, it is important that you are aware of the information a person has the right to know at the time of their diagnosis. The General Medical Council in their Good Medical Practice Guide (2006) states that a person has the right to know: their diagnosis, prognosis and timescale, treatment options, the outcome of treatment, side-effects of any treatment and the cost of the treatment options where relevant. During this initial consultation it is unlikely that the person will hear all that is being said and will leave with questions to ask. Adler et al. (1989) recognise the impact of physical and psychological noise on communication: physical noise could include the environment that the interaction is taking place in and sensory impairment, and psychological noise could be the distractions, fears and preconceptions, of both the patient and the nurse, that are brought to the situation.

Activity 1.4   *Critical thinking*

Case scenario: Angela

Following the birth of her son Charlie six months ago, Angela (aged 28) has been feeling tired and has been experiencing muscular aches and pains. Initially she put these down to being a 'new mum'; however she was persuaded to see her General Practitioner (GP) by her husband James. She has been undergoing a series of investigations and she is attending an appointment with her consultant to find out the results of the investigations. Both James and Charlie have come along to the appointment with Angela.

You are on placement in the outpatient department, and the consultant has asked that your mentor sits in on Angela's consultation – you go in with her. It is during this consultation that Angela is given her diagnosis of RRMS.

- What physical and psychological noise may impact on Angela and James's ability to take on board information?
- What could you do to minimise the impact of these?

A brief outline answer is given at the end of the chapter.

Activity 1.4 demonstrates the need for ongoing communication for people diagnosed with an LTC and their family. You should provide relevant information in an appropriate format and recap as necessary to ensure that the information has been understood by the person and their family. The impact of living with an LTC goes beyond the point of diagnosis and stays with the person and their family as their condition progresses. It is important therefore to remember that 'noise' may be present at other times during a person's health journey. A person living with an LTC will feel the impact of their diagnosis in all areas of their life, physically, psychologically and socially. The remainder of this section will discuss the physical and psychological impact of living with an LTC. The social impact will be discussed in Chapter 3 in relation to **determinants of health** and public health.

The physical impact of living with an LTC

Many of the physical effects of living with an LTC are condition-specific. There is not scope in this section to outline the altered pathology and the signs and symptoms of all LTCs, therefore the remainder of this section will outline the altered physiology and the main signs and symptoms of the following LTCs: asthma, chronic heart failure, epilepsy, prostate cancer, HIV and dementia. Information on the altered physiology and the signs and symptoms of coronary heart disease, rheumatoid arthritis and Parkinson's disease can be found in Activity 5.1 in Chapter 5.

Asthma

Asthma is an inflammatory lung condition where the airways in the lungs are hyper-responsive to a range of irritants. Asthma can be described as being intrinsic, where no specific irritant can be found, or extrinsic, where an identifiable irritant is present. Such irritants include smoke, pollen, household allergens, e.g. dust mites, medication, e.g. non-steroidal anti-inflammatory drugs and infection, e.g. upper respiratory tract. When exposed to an irritant, the muscle in the airways contracts, and the membranes shrink, resulting in a narrowing of the airways. As the airway narrows, the flow of air to the lungs is disrupted, resulting in an 'asthma attack' where the person experiences wheeze, chest tightness, shortness of breath and coughing (Clinical Knowledge Summaries (CKS), 2007). As well as narrowing of the airways the irritants cause inflammation of the membranes and excessive production of mucus (Lorig et al., 2006). This inflammatory response is reversible; however, if it is not managed correctly it can lead to complication such as respiratory failure, **status asthmasticus** and irreversible damage of the airways. Asthma can also lead to fatigue, resulting in time off work or school (CKS, 2007).

Chronic heart failure

Chronic heart failure (CHF) can be associated with previous myocardial infarction or other cardiovascular conditions, e.g. hypertension. It can be caused by either high or low cardiac output. High cardiac output is where the heart is working a normal or increased rate but the requirements of the body are more than the heart can supply, e.g. anaemia, hyperthyroidism. Low cardiac output is caused by a reduction in the function of the heart and is due to the following (Simon et al., 2002):

- increased pre-loading of the heart, e.g. fluid overload or mitral regurgitation;
- failure of the pumping mechanism of the heart, e.g. ischaemic heart disease;
- inadequate heart rate, e.g. use of beta blockers;
- arrhythmia, e.g. atrial fibrillation;
- excessive overloading, e.g. hypertension.

When discussing CHF it is common to use the terms 'right heart failure' and 'left heart failure', resulting in differing signs and symptoms due to the nature of the heart failure. Right heart failure is usually associated with congestion of the veins throughout the person's body while left heart failure is usually associated with congestion of the pulmonary veins (CKS, 2009a). In right heart failure a person can experience the following: ankle oedema, abdominal discomfort due to liver distension, fatigue and nausea and anorexia. People with left heart failure can experience the following: shortness of breath (on exertion and **orthopnea**), fatigue, reduced exercise tolerance and nocturnal cough (Simon et al., 2002; CKS, 2009a).

Epilepsy

Epilepsy is a neurological condition that is caused by abnormal bursts of electrical activity in the brain due to increased neural activity. This presents as a **transient** disturbance of consciousness, behaviour, emotion, motor function or sensation (CKS, 2009b). These episodes are called epileptic seizures and can last from a few seconds to a few minutes. Epilepsy is not a single condition; therefore the symptoms occurring during a seizure will vary depending on the part of the brain affected by the increase in neural activity (Drennan and Goodman, 2007).

- Focal epilepsy – this involves one part of the body; seizures will start in that part and then progress to other parts of the body, becoming generalised (Jacksonian epilepsy).
- Grand mal epilepsy – this presents as a generalised seizure with sudden onset of **tonic** contraction of the muscles and **clonic** convulsions occurring on both sides of the body and at the same time. Following the seizure the person is usually unconscious and takes time to recover.
- Petit mal epilepsy – this is characterised by a pause in speech or activity, with the person being unaware of the episode.
- Myoclonic epilepsy – this is a variation of petit mal epilepsy, resulting in **atonic** drop attacks.
- Temporal lobe epilepsy – during seizures the person may remain conscious and can experience sensory, emotional and cognitive changes, including oral and auditory hallucinations.

Status epilepticus is a complication of epilepsy and occurs when a seizure lasts more than 30 minutes, or a person has successive convulsions where they do not recover consciousness between the seizures (CKS, 2009b). Treatment aims to stop seizures from occurring; however, should this not be possible the aim is to reduce their frequency and severity. Epilepsy can have a significant impact on the day-to-day life of a person, e.g. people with epilepsy must be seizure-free for one year before they are able to hold a driving licence (CKS, 2009b). Therefore providing information regarding epilepsy, the day-to-day management and how to manage seizures increases a person's sense of control and minimises the stigma attached to the condition.

Prostate cancer

Prostate cancer is the most common cancer in men: more than 34,000 men are diagnosed with prostate cancer each year (Cancer Research UK, 2010). The prostate gland is found only in men; it lies just beneath the bladder and is normally the size of a walnut and is divided into two lobes. The urethra runs through the middle of the prostate: the main function of the prostate is to produce fluid which enriches and protects sperm. The growth and function of the prostate gland depends on the production of testosterone, a hormone produced in the testes. Prostate cancer develops due to the formation of abnormal cells in the prostate gland. These cells cause the prostate to increase in size: as prostate cancer is a slow-growing cancer, in the early stages of the disease there may be no symptoms. Symptoms of local prostate cancer include urinary retention and haematuria; frequency of micturition and urgency can be present (CKS, 2005). As the cancer spreads the person may experience symptoms such as weight loss, bone pain and fatigue (Simon et al., 2002).

Human immunodeficiency virus (HIV)

HIV is a retrovirus that causes infections; the long term symptoms of the condition and the condition itself develop slowly over a period of time. Two species of HIV have been identified: HIV-1, which is highly contagious and transmittable and is found throughout the world; and HIV-2, which is less contagious and transmittable and is predominately found in West Africa and Portugal (CKS, 2010a). HIV affects a person's immune system: HIV infects cells in the immune system, predominately CD4 cells. These cells are called t-helper cells and are crucial to activating cell immunity. The virus binds itself to the CD4 receptor and infects the CD4 cell with its ribonucleic acid (RNA). Due to its specific properties RNA is able to convert the viral RNA into DNA, which is then incorporated into the person's DNA. The virus then lies dormant until the CD4 cells are activated due to infection. When this occurs, new HIV enzymes are produced; these mature viruses then detach from the walls of the CD4 cell, enter the blood stream and infect other cells in the body (CKS, 2010a). In HIV the virus is present in all cell-containing body fluid, e.g. blood, semen, vaginal secretions, breast milk, pleural effusions and cerebrospinal fluid. Therefore transmission can occur when infected body fluid enters another person's blood stream, e.g. needle-stick injury and sexual activity. HIV leaves a person susceptible to infection, resulting in tiredness, pyrexia, and joint and muscle pain. Some of these symptoms can be mild and mistaken for other conditions, such as the common cold. HIV can progress into acquired immune deficiency syndrome (AIDS). Diagnosis is made on the basis of a low CD4 count, below 200, and if an AIDS-defining clinical condition is present, e.g. Kaposi's sarcoma, recurrent pneumonia, ongoing herpes simplex infection for more than one month (CKS, 2010a). At this point, due to the damage to the immune system, a person may be experiencing night sweats, weight loss, shortness of breath and pyrexia. Specialist support will be able to address the wide range of psychological, emotional, social and physical needs a person living with HIV may have.

Dementia

Dementia is a **syndrome** that occurs due to damage to a person's brain, resulting in many problems, such as memory loss, although their level of consciousness is not affected (Simon et al.,

2002). Most of these syndromes progress gradually over a period of years; a person's ability to manage their activities of daily living (ADL) independently is affected by their declining memory and cognitive ability.

The symptoms of dementia occur in three areas (CKS, 2010b).

1. Cognitive dysfunction – this results in a person experiencing many problems, e.g. language (both speech and written), memory and orientation to time, place and person.
2. Psychiatric and behavioural problems – these include personality changes, reduced emotional control (emotionally labile) and agitation.
3. Difficulties with ADLs – areas that are affected include driving, personal care and shopping.

The incidence of dementia in the population increases with age; conventionally a person developing dementia under the age of 65 is classed as having early or young-onset dementia. The most common causes of dementia are listed below (CKS, 2010b).

- Alzheimer's disease accounts for approximately 50% of all cases of dementia. It is caused by degenerative changes in the cerebral cortex, resulting in pathological changes to the structure and chemistry of a person's brain. The cortex of the brain atrophies, and amyloid (fibrous protein) plaques form on and around the neurones. Neurones affected by this have reduced production of acetylcholine (a neurotransmitter involved in learning, memory and mood). Initially a person experiences memory lapses, e.g. forgetting names and places. As the disease progresses, symptoms like problems with language and mood changes (depression and agitation) occur.
- Vascular dementia accounts for about 25% of dementia cases and is sometimes called vascular cognitive impairment. Damage to the brain is as a result of cerebrovascular disease, including cerebrovascular accident (CVA), small undetected CVAs (multi-infarct) or ongoing changes in the small cerebral blood vessels (subcortical dementia). In this type of dementia each cerebrovascular event causes an increase in the person's symptoms; these include personality changes, some focal neurological deficit and apathy.

Management of dementia includes providing the person and their carer with strategies to manage their memory loss, social and carer support and management of presenting symptoms, e.g. agitation, sleep disturbance (Simon et al., 2002).

Activity 1.5   *Evidence-based practice and research*

Using the scenarios outlined in Activity 1.3 for Angela, Andrew and Frazer, briefly outline the altered physiology and the main signs and symptoms of:

- RRMS;
- COPD;
- Type 1 diabetes.

Some useful resources:

- your preferred applied anatomy and physiology text books;
- www.cks.nhs.uk/home – this is a useful website for healthcare professionals working

continued overleaf...

continued...

in primary care, and provides evidence-based information on managing common conditions seen in primary care;

- www.patient.co.uk/ – this comprehensive website contains information on many health conditions.

A brief outline answer is given at the end of the chapter.

Activity 1.5 demonstrates the profound effect on the day-to-day life of the person that the physical symptoms of an LTC can have. Many of these, such as pain and fatigue, can be mentally exhausting to live with too, and can have a negative psychological impact on the person's mental wellbeing. Depression is known to occur in approximately 20% of people who are living with an LTC (NICE, 2009a).

The psychological impact of living with an LTC

People living with a condition such as Type 2 diabetes, hypertension, CVA, COPD or end-stage renal disease are two to three times more likely to develop depression than people who are in good physical health (Haddad, 2010). It is known that living with an LTC can both cause and increase a person's depression. This **comorbidity** adversely affects the course and outcome of both their underlying LTC and their overlying mental health condition. For example, a person living with rheumatoid arthritis who is experiencing pain and reduced functional ability has an increased risk of developing depression, which may, in turn, increase their pain and distress, creating a cycle of symptoms (NICE, 2009a). There is also evidence to suggest that depression can increase the likelihood of a person developing conditions such as heart disease (Nicholson et al., 2006) or Type 2 diabetes (Mezuk et al., 2008). Diagnosing and managing depression is important for the person living with an LTC. It is known that depression has a negative effect on a person's health outcome, their level of disability and how well they utilise available resources (Care Services Improvement Partnership (CSIP), 2006).

A formal diagnosis of depression is made using either the ICD-10 classification system or the DSM-IV system, with symptoms having been present for at least two weeks and evident on most days. When using these systems there are some key symptoms that need to be present for a diagnosis of depression to be made. These are: low mood, loss of interest and pleasure or loss of energy (NICE, 2009b). However, for people living with an LTC identifying depression can be challenging as many of the physical symptoms of depression, (e.g. fatigue, insomnia and reduced appetite) may also be related to the LTC and its treatment. So it is important that you are alert to the possibility of a person developing depression. Although you will not be involved in diagnosing depression, your knowledge and understanding of an individual may alert you to changes in their mood that could indicate depression. NICE (2009a) recommends the Two-Question Screen Tool for people with an LTC who may have depression.

1. During the last month, have you often been bothered by feeling down, depressed or hopeless?

2. During recentmonths, have you often been bothered by having little interest or pleasure in doing things?

As these questions link to the key symptoms required for a diagnosis of depression to be made this screening tool has excellent sensitivity (Haddad, 2010). If a person answers yes to one or both questions a more detailed assessment for depression should be undertaken. In situations where communication is difficult, e.g. sensory impairment or learning disability, a visual analogue like the distress thermometer can be used (NICE, 2009a). Using a picture of a thermometer and a scale of 0 to 10 it uses a single question screen: *how distressed have you been during the past week on a scale of 0 to 10?* If any significant level of distress is identified, a score of 4 or more, this should be reported and investigated further. If necessary a referral to specialist services, e.g. community learning disability services, should be made. Once a diagnosis of depression has been made, appropriate treatment and management is required. Both NICE (2009a) and CSIP (2006) recommend the use of the stepped care framework, as outlined in Table 1.2.

Who is responsible for care?	In this situation	What do they do?
Acute wards	Risk to life	Medication, in-patient care
Mental health specialists	Treatment resistance and frequent recurrences	Medication, complex psychological interventions
Primary care mental health worker, GP, GP with special interest, counsellor, social worker, psychologist	Moderate or severe disorders	Medication, brief psychological interventions, support groups
GP, practice nurse, practice counsellor	Mild disorders	Active review: self-help, cognitive behavioural therapy, exercise
Primary care team	Recognition	Watchful waiting and assessment

Table 1.2: Stepped care for depression in LTCs
(Sources: NICE, 2009a; CSIP, 2006)

Activity 1.6   *Reflection*

Reflecting back on your recent clinical experience, can you identify a situation where it would have been appropriate to ask the questions in the Two-Question Screen Tool described above?

If these questions had been asked would the person's response to these have altered your care? If so, how?

As the answers will be based on your own observations there is no outline answer at the end of this chapter.

Many people find discussing mental health issues uncomfortable; this applies to the person with the LTC and the healthcare professionals involved in their care. Activity 1.6 will have highlighted that in some cases addressing mental health issues relies on you having the confidence to discuss mental health issues with those in your care. The information in Chapter 2 of this book can be used to support you to develop effective therapeutic relationships, fostering a relationship that is open and non-judgemental. Developing trust in this way encourages those in your care to communicate their hopes and fears and can assist you in recognising changes in a person's mental health.

Care across the lifespan: the transition from child to adult services

An estimated 15% of children under the age of five and 20% of children between the ages of five and 15 are living with an LTC (DH, 2005; Drennan and Goodman, 2007). Many of these children are living into adulthood and require continuing support and care during their adult years to enable them to successfully manage their condition in order to live as healthy and as independent a life as possible. It is important therefore that you gain an understanding of the role of transition within the care and management of children living with an LTC. This will enable you to work with child health professionals and better support those in your care. Adolescence is a time of change for all young people, with many social and psychological changes taking place, e.g. peer pressure, pushing boundaries and increasing responsibilities. However, young people living with an LTC face particular challenges. This is recognised in standard 4 of *The National Service Framework for Children, Young People and Maternity Services: Core Standards* (DH, 2004). Here the need for age-appropriate services that are responsive to a young person's changing needs as they grow into adulthood is emphasised. Transition is described as a process and not as an event and should be planned for early:

> *A purposeful, planned process that addresses the medical, psychosocial and educational/vocational needs of adolescents and young adults with chronic physical and medical conditions as they move from child-centred to adult-orientated health care system.*

> (DH, 2006, page 14)

Activity 1.7   *Reflection*

Reflecting back on your recent clinical experience and considering the information above, what is your experience of how care has been managed and provided for adolescents? What were some of the challenges faced by both the young adult and their family?

As the answers will be based on your own observations there is no outline answer at the end of this chapter.

In Activity 1.7 you may have identified that in some cases the care and management of adolescents could have been more effectively managed. It is known that organised transition programmes benefit young people and their families in many ways: improved follow up, better disease control and improved documentation, resulting in improved communication and care. There is also evidence to suggest that poor transition and a lack of follow-up leads a young person to disengage from health services, and this can have a negative impact on their health (DH, 2008c). A recent report by New Philanthropy Capital (McGrath and Yeowart, 2009) noted that many of the needs of young people during transition were not being met by healthcare services but were being met by charities instead. Within the UK the charity Contact a Family (www.cafamily.org.uk) provides region-based information for families where a child has an LTC:

* *Preparing for adult life and transition: information for families, England and Wales*;
* *Preparing for adult life and transition – Northern Ireland*;
* *Preparing for adult life and transition – Scotland.*

In recognition of this, the DH (2008c) aims to build on areas of good practice to further support the transition process by placing the child at the centre of the process and planning for transition early. The DH (2008c) recommends that transition from child to adult services should begin when a child is approximately 13 years and support should continue until they are 25 years old. This is to tie in with an age when young people are already receiving advice regarding education and career choices. This approach allows the young person to plan their healthcare transition alongside planning for their future career and independence. Transition should be coordinated by a key worker from child health services, and, if possible, a designated key worker from adult services to promote continuity of care during the transition period. There are many strategies that can be used to support transition planning.

Health transition plans (DH, 2008c)

Working with appropriate members of the healthcare team, health transition plans are developed by the young person and focus on what they can do to stay healthy, minimise their health need and maximise their independence. This collaborative approach allows the young person to identify their needs and work with healthcare professionals to write up an action plan to meet these needs. By engaging the young person in the early stages there is the opportunity to increase their feelings of control and empowerment and to develop their self-management skills (DH2008c). A health transition plan should:

* assist the young person to become more knowledgeable and confident in making decisions that impact on their health and healthcare needs, e.g. action planning and self-management;
* support the young person in understanding their LTC and how to minimise the impact of their LTC on their future health and wellbeing, e.g. health education and health promotion;
* promote the sharing of information, where appropriate, between relevant health and social care services, e.g. health records being held by the young person;
* address transition in the context of the young person's life, taking into account all the person's needs, e.g. education.

As well as focusing on the needs of the young person, the health transition plan should also focus on the young person's strengths and include all areas of the person's life. There should be a clear focus on promoting health and wellbeing and what is required to achieve this. The young person's physical, emotional (including sexual health) and social health should be assessed along with their ability for self-care, including any aids and adaptations required. The young person's ability to participate in the medical management of their LTC should also be assessed, including administration of medication. In the broader context of the young person's life their education, training and leisure requirements should also be assessed, with the aim being to maximise the young person's independence (DH, 2008c). For the parents of a young person the transition of care from child to adult health services can often cause anxiety. This is in part due to the increasing independence of the young person, who may now be making their own decisions, resulting in the parent feeling excluded (Flemming et al., 2002). It is important therefore that transition planning incorporates not just the needs of the young person but the needs of the whole family. If the young person and their family work effectively with child health services early in the transition process, this will enable the young person to develop the required knowledge and skills to successfully manage their LTC into their adult life and will support the family in their changing roles.

Conclusion

Having read this chapter and worked through the activities you will have developed your knowledge and skills in relation to the impact of LTCs across the lifespan. How you use this new knowledge will depend on where you are working and your roles and responsibilities. As a nurse you can improve your knowledge of the impact of LTCs across the lifespan in many ways. By increasing your understanding of how the care and management of LTCs is delivered, you will be able to liaise with other members of the healthcare team to provide an appropriate level of care. You can better support people living with an LTC by developing your knowledge and understanding of the physical and psychological impact of living with a variety of LTCs. This will enable you to provide care that directly meets the needs of the person and will enable you to plan appropriate care for future needs. By working with your child health colleagues you will be able to support young people during a crucial time in their healthcare journey, ensuring that they gain the necessary knowledge and skills to manage their LTC into adulthood.

Chapter summary

This chapter has provided you with an overview of the impact of LTCs across the lifespan. It has outlined the incidence of LTCs in both adults and children and the impact this has on healthcare services and their design. In outlining the physical and psychological impact of living with an LTC it has identified the importance of having a good understanding of the signs and symptoms of a variety of LTCs. It has emphasised the need for timely and focused transition planning to ensure young people do not disengage from healthcare services at an important time in their health journey. Specific strategies in relation to recognising depression in people with an LTC and during transition from child to adult services have been discussed and related to your clinical practice.

Activities: brief outline answers

Activity 1.1: Critical thinking (page 7)

The information in this table is based on information from the article by Holman and Lorig (2002).

	Acute conditions	**LTCs**
Onset	Abrupt, for example, appendicitis, meningitis, pneumonia.	Generally gradually over a period of time, though some conditions can progress rapidly, e.g. motor neurone disease
Duration	Limited duration, once over the initial episode. Though may result in some long term implication, e.g. cognitive impairment following meningitis	Present over a long period of time, with no definite end point
Cause	Usually has a single cause, e.g. bacterial infection	May be due to lifestyle factors, genetics or cause may not be known. One LTC may result in other symptoms, e.g. Type 1 diabetes may result in autonomic neuropathy
Diagnosis and prognosis	A diagnosis is usually made quickly and accurately	Diagnosis can take time, difficult to predict the outcome, can lead to uncertainty
Therapeutic interventions	Usually effective in managing the condition, e.g. targeted use of antibiotics for bacterial infection	Often only able to manage symptoms, side-effects present, e.g. triple therapy for HIV can cause fatigue and gastrointestinal upset
Outcome	Cure is possible	No cure is available
Uncertainty	Minimal uncertainty is present in most cases, though for conditions like meningitis the impact may last longer	High levels of uncertainty due to complexities of managing the condition and increasing symptoms
Knowledge	Generally healthcare professionals are knowledgeable and provide information; patients can lack knowledge of condition	Both the person living with the LTC and the professionals involved in their care share their knowledge

Some LTCs: asthma, arthritis (osteo and rheumatoid), diabetes (Types 1 and 2), epilepsy, some cancers, chronic obstructive pulmonary disease (COPD), motor neurone disease (MND), cerebrovascular accident (CVA), dementia, depression, psoriasis, coronary heart disease (CHD), HIV, Parkinson's disease, muscular dystrophy, hepatitis (B, C and D), chronic kidney disease, Crohn's disease, diverticulitis, cerebral palsy, cystic fibrosis, traumatic head injury, sensory impairment, e.g. deafness.

Activity 1.2 Reflection (page 8)

Over the course of his life it is likely that Ali and his family will have come into contact with the following health and social care professionals and services.

- Primary healthcare team: GP and practice nurse for ongoing monitoring of his hypertension, regular blood tests, monitoring of transplant and health promotion regarding smoking cessation. Support from the CAPD nurse and team during his CAPD treatment, e.g. importance of fluid balance, hygiene and maintenance of system. Access and support to the renal outreach team regarding home dialysis, including education and training. Access to community pharmacy for medication throughout his life, may require this to be delivered to his house in the later stages of his illness. District nursing input required as his health deteriorated, e.g. pain relief, support from social services regarding personal care, assessment and provision of equipment from occupational therapy, e.g. walking aid, hospital bed at home. Palliative care services, both for Ali and his family.
- Secondary care services: regular review by outpatient services, renal consultant and renal nurse specialist. In-patient care for insertion of CAPD catheter and both renal transplants including care in high-dependency or intensive care. Follow-up care from renal/transplant outreach team, e.g. psychological support. In-patient services will be required for Ali's dialysis; he may require transport to and from his local renal unit.

This does not include access to services as a result of an emergency or for aspects of care not related to his kidney disease.

Ali's condition may affect his family in the following ways:

- changing of roles and responsibilities within the family, especially for Ali's wife as his condition deteriorates;
- impact of Ali's condition on his children, medical equipment at home, visits to hospitals;
- making changes to the house to accommodate Ali's CAPD, home dialysis and in the later stages equipment needed to enable Ali to stay at home;
- carer responsibilities for both his wife and children, especially as they grow older; for people on home dialysis it is important that they have support and someone able to deal with emergencies;
- financial implications, cost of any adaptations, reduction in family income if Ali is not able to work;
- increase in stress for all family members, including the realisation that Ali will die due to the advanced nature of his disease.

Activity 1.3: Decision making (page 11)

Angela – supported self-care/management; Andrew – disease/care management; Frazer – supported self-care/management though is accessing some disease/care management.

Activity 1.4: Critical thinking (page 13)

Physical noise
- There may be noise coming in from outside the room.
- Charlie may be crying/babbling.

Psychological noise
- They may be distracted by Charlie.
- They may have heard the words 'multiple sclerosis' and not listened to anything after that.
- They may be worried about each other.

Physical noise
- Minimise disturbances, ensure phones are redirected, ask other staff to keep the area quiet.
- Offer to take Charlie out of the room while they are having their consultation.

Psychological noise
- Spend some time ensuring Charlie is happy and settled, offer to take Charlie out of the room for the remainder of the consultation.
- Observe their verbal and non-verbal communication for signs of confusion and distress. Note at what point in the consultation this was at – it may be necessary to go over information later. Listen to their questions/comments – they will provide you with useful information as to how much they have heard/understood and what may need to be recapped on.

Activity 1.5: Evidence-based practice and research (page 17)

RRMS

This is the most common type of multiple sclerosis (MS) and is characterised by numerous relapses and remissions. Relapses are periods of time where symptoms are worse; these are often followed by periods of remission where symptoms disappear or improve. Relapses may last for days, weeks or even months. During a relapse a person may experience new symptoms or may have a recurrence of previous symptoms (Drennan and Goodman, 2007).

MS is a neurological condition affecting a person's central nervous system (CNS). Nerve fibres in the CNS are surrounded and protected by myelin; this substance insulates the nerve fibres, allowing messages to travel quickly and smoothly within the CNS.

MS is an autoimmune condition: a person's body mistakes part of their own body as a foreign body and attacks it. In the case of MS it is the myelin that is attacked and damaged. This damage causes demyelination, where the myelin covering the nerve fibres is reduced and scars called lesions develop. Demyelination disrupts the messages travelling along the nerve fibres, e.g. slowing them down.

The symptoms of MS depend on the part of the CNS affected but can include fatigue, continence problems, visual disturbances, muscle spasm and pain, and emotional problems such as depression (CKS, no date; Drennan and Goodman, 2007). Depression is common in people with MS; it is present in as many as 29% of all cases.

COPD

This is a lung condition that is characterised by airflow obstruction; this is usually progressive with the obstruction being due to a combination of airway diseases, chronic bronchitis and emphysema. It is associated with an abnormal inflammatory response of the lungs to noxious stimuli, e.g. cigarette smoke (Drennan and Goodman, 2007).

Chronic bronchitis is clinically defined as a persistent cough with sputum production for at least three months of the year for two consecutive years. Cigarette smoke causes **hyperplasia** and **hypertrophy** of the mucus-secreting glands found in the large airways, e.g. bronchioles. As a result of this a person's small airways become obstructed with mucus plugs and oedema, resulting in a reduction of the action of the cilia, preventing the movement of mucus from the small to large airways to be expectorated. This reduces the level of gaseous exchange in the lungs.

Emphysema is the permanent enlargement of the air space **distal** to the terminal bronchiole as a result of alveolar septal destruction. As distal airways are held open by the alveolar septa this destruction causes the airways to collapse, resulting in obstruction. As the alveolar walls are destroyed, **bullae** form, and destruction of the parenchyma (gas exchange tissue) leads to a reduction in perfusion of oxygen from the lungs to the blood stream (Patel and Gwilt, 2008). A person with COPD may present with breathlessness on exertion, chronic cough, frequent infections, fatigue and weight loss.

Type 1 diabetes

This condition occurs when a person's body does not produce insulin and often develops in teenage years and almost always before the age of 40. Insulin is a hormone produced by the pancreas: in Type 1 diabetes autoimmune responses damage the beta cells of the islet cells in the pancreas. This results in a lack of insulin or no insulin being produced (Simon et al., 2002). Normally insulin is secreted by the pancreas as the level of glucose in the blood stream increases, usually associated with digestion of food, and is responsible for moving glucose from the blood stream to the cells to be converted into energy.

In Type 1 diabetes this does not happen and blood glucose levels rise (hyperglycaemia); this inefficient use of glucose results in a person experiencing increased thirst (glucose leaks into the urine, causing the kidneys to excrete water), weight loss (though appetite often increases as the body tries to metabolise energy from food) and tiredness (CKS, no date). Over time even mildly elevated levels of glucose in the blood stream can cause damage to the blood vessels, resulting in atheroma, visual disturbances due to damage to the small vessels of the retina and poor circulation, both peripheral and central.

Further reading

Department of Health (2008c) *Transition: Moving on Well.* London: Department of Health.
This includes an example transition health plan and useful information about multidisciplinary transition planning.

Drennan, V and Goodman C (2007) *Oxford Handbook of Primary Care and Community Nursing.* Oxford: Oxford University Press.
Contains a useful chapter on the care of people with LTCs, including signs and symptoms and management

Useful websites

www.cks.nhs.uk/home
A reliable source of practical evidence-based information on a range of common conditions managed in primary care.

www.cafamily.org.uk
This is a UK-wide charity providing information and support for families who are living with a disabled child.

www.patient.co.uk
A site providing comprehensive health information similar to that provided by GPs and nurses to patients during consultations.

www.transitionpathway.co.uk
The transition pathway is a resource pack that can be used by anyone who is involved in supporting young people in the transition to adulthood.

Chapter 2
The therapeutic relationship in long term conditions

• • *continued...* •

6. People can trust the newly registered graduate nurse to engage therapeutically and actively listen to their needs and concerns, responding using skills that are helpful, providing information that is clear, accurate, meaningful and free from jargon.

By the first progression point:

1. Communicates effectively both orally and in writing, so that the meaning is always clear.

By the second progression point:

6. Uses strategies to enhance communication and remove barriers to effective communication, minimising risk to people from lack of or poor communication.

By entry to the register:

11. Is proactive and creative in enhancing communication and understanding.

12. Uses the skills of active listening and questioning, paraphrasing and reflection to support a therapeutic intervention.

Chapter aims

After reading this chapter you will be able to:

- identify and describe the components of the therapeutic relationship;
- explain the importance of engaging in a therapeutic relationship with people living with a long term condition and, if required, their carer and family;
- understand the components of emotional intelligence (EI) and its relevance to the care and management of those living with a long term condition;
- recognise the importance of ensuring person-focused communication in the care and management of those living with a long term condition.

Introduction

Cure sometimes: treat often: comfort always.

(Hippocrates 460–370 BC)

I will remember that there is art to medicine as well as science, and that warmth, sympathy, and understanding may outweigh the surgeon's knife or the chemist's drug.

(Hippocratic oath – modern version)

Engaging in, developing and maintaining caring and compassionate therapeutic relationships is at the heart of effective nursing care. Doing this allows you, the nurse, to provide person-centred, individualised nursing care. The Nursing and Midwifery Council (NMC) places therapeutic relationships and communication at the heart of *The Code: standards of conduct, performance and ethics for nurses and midwives* (NMC, 2008).

Those living with a long term condition (LTC) can be in contact with healthcare professionals on many occasions and over a long period of time; this may take the form of a review with their practice nurse or when receiving in-patient care due to an exacerbation. At all stages of a person's journey a key element of their care is your ability to foster holistic person-centred care, promoting **concordance** with treatment and management regimes, foster **autonomy** in managing their own condition and increasing their satisfaction with their care. The development and maintenance of a person-centred therapeutic relationship is central to this: this may involve not only forming a relationship with the individual but also their family and carers. For those living with an LTC, and those caring for them, it may not be the 'what' of the treatment (e.g. the intravenous antibiotics for a chest infection) the person remembers but the 'how' of the treatment. 'How' the treatment was delivered, were they listened to, was the treatment explained to them, was there a friendly face there, did they feel understood? To support you in your delivery of 'meaningful' care to those living with an LTC this chapter will assist you in your development of the knowledge and skills required to successfully develop an effective therapeutic relationship with those requiring your care. In order to do this the chapter will help you to develop your knowledge, skills and attributes in relation to understanding what a therapeutic relationship is, emotional intelligence and the relationship you have with carers. Some specific communication strategies useful when caring for those living with an LTC are also addressed.

Case study: Bill

Bill and his wife were struggling to manage his long term conditions (angina and COPD); through working with Bill's community matron they have become more actively involved in the management of Bill's cardiac and lung problems. Both Bill and his wife have regained their confidence and are now able to live more independently. Bill told his story to Patient Voices, a programme founded to support the telling of individuals' stories of health and social care. Figure 2.1 is a word cloud of Bill's story, allowing you to see the words that appeared most frequently.

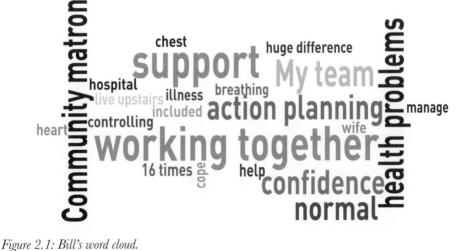

Figure 2.1: Bill's word cloud.
(Source: Patient Voices website, reproduced with permission.)

To listen to Bill's story follow the link: ***www.patientvoices.org.uk/flv/0029pv384.htm.***

An effective therapeutic relationship enables us to *work together* as a *team* with individuals and their carers to *support* them to *manage* their condition and improve their *confidence* in their ability to *manage* their condition.

Policy review

Before we go on to consider the therapeutic relationship in more detail, it is useful to consider the broader context of the policy around this subject. Both the therapeutic relationships and placing the individual at the heart of the nursing process have been central to many recent health publications in the UK. In England the Department of Health (DH) published the *National Service Framework for Older People* (2001) and the *National Service Framework for Long Term Conditions* (2005a). Standard two of the *National Service Framework for Older People* focuses on person-centred care, ensuring that older people are listened to, are able to make informed choices and are involved in all decisions about their needs and care. This is echoed in the *National Service Framework for Long Term Conditions* (DH, 2005a), quality requirement 1: a person-centred service; the aim of this requirement is to ensure that those living with an LTC are able to make informed decisions about their care and treatment and, where possible, to manage their conditions themselves. In Scotland the Scottish Government Health Delivery Directorate Improvement Support Team published *Long Term Conditions Collaborative: High Impact Changes* (2009); high impact change 2 focused on the active involvement of the person, and carer, in their care planning and ongoing care with the person's needs the focus for any care planning. In Northern Ireland the Long Term Conditions Alliance Northern Ireland (2008), responding to the proposed changes in health and social care in Northern Ireland, put forward by the Department of Health, Social Services and Public Safety, supported the principle that the delivery of services should be focused on the needs of the person and carers and that those living with an LTC have a key role to play in the planning and delivery of their care. In Wales the publication *Designed to Improve Health and Management of Chronic Conditions in Wales: An integrated model and framework* (Department of Health and Social Services (DHSS), 2007) again placed value on the role of the person and carer as active partners in the planning of their care. To ensure that the focus on any interaction is clearly centred on the individual, the development of an effective therapeutic relationship between nurse and individual is fundamental.

While these publications relate to the management of long term conditions within the UK in England, other, more general, Department of Health publications focused on all service provision within healthcare and the need for person-centred, personalised services (DH, 2006, 2010). This ethos is summed up in the latest Department of Health publication, *Equity and Excellence: liberating the NHS*: with the principle, *no decision about me without me* (DH, 2010, page 3).

The therapeutic relationship

> *The therapeutic relationship is grounded in an interpersonal process that occurs between the nurse and patient. It is a purposeful, goal-directed relationship that is directed at advancing the best interests and outcome of the patient.*
>
> (Registered Nurses Association of Ontario, 2002, page 13)

So what is the therapeutic relationship and why is it important to nursing? In 2003 the Royal College of Nursing (RCN) set out a definition of nursing as being:

The use of clinical judgement in the provision of care to enable people to improve, maintain or recover health, to cope with health problems, and to achieve the best possible quality of life, whatever their disease or disability, until death.

(Royal College of Nursing, 2003, page 3)

Inherent within this definition is the notion of enabling. While the above quote emphasises clinical judgement if nurses are to truly enable those in their care, and provide person-centred care that meets and addresses their needs, then the development and maintenance of an effective therapeutic relationship is essential. An effective therapeutic relationship allows you to ensure that the focus of your nursing interventions is on the whole person and their response to the situation (RCN, 2003). To do this, engaging in and developing a therapeutic relationship allows you to recognise the uniqueness of the person and its success depends on your ability to make and maintain personal/professional relationships with those in your care (Foster and Hawkins, 2005). The characteristics that define a successful therapeutic relationship (Chilton et al., 2004) include:

• maintaining appropriate boundaries;
• meeting the needs of the person;
• promoting the autonomy of the person;
• ensuring a positive experience for the person.

We will now look in more detail at each of these.

Maintaining appropriate boundaries

Within the therapeutic relationship the maintenance of boundaries is crucial: boundaries define and manage expectation, and they ensure all parties are clear about what can reasonably be expected from each other. The Nursing and Midwifery Council (NMC, 2010) states that nurses must respect professional boundaries at all times, therefore it is your responsibility to ensure that appropriate professional boundaries are maintained. For nurses involved in the care and management of those with LTCs the nature of their relationship may vary: specialist nurses may be involved in delivering short term interventions, while community matrons may be involved in longer term care and care planning. These types of interactions will involve different levels of relationship building. Those involved in shorter interventions may focus on the intervention and its success while those involved in longer term care may be more likely to emphasise the development of a connected relationship, where you view the individual as a person first and foremost (Morse, 1991).

• The development of a therapeutic relationship is not without its challenges, and for the majority of nurses boundaries are maintained, allowing for the delivery of more person-focused and person-led care. However, given the ongoing nature of the therapeutic relationship in the management of LTCs, there may be the potential for boundaries to 'blur'. Recognising situations when this may happen will assist you in maintaining professional boundaries within the therapeutic relationship; it is about being personable rather than personal, possessing and using effective communication and interpersonal skills while maintaining professional boundaries. Table 2.1 outlines some useful questions (Chilton et al., 2004) to ask yourself to promote appropriate boundaries.

Question	Response
Is the focus of this relationship on the person and their needs?	If the answer is no, use the questions below to ensure that the focus remains on the person and their needs: • Have you undertaken a person-focused assessment? • Were you listening to the person and using this information to plan their care? • Have you let what you believe is right for the person influence their plan of care?
Is this person beginning to rely on me too much?	If the answer is yes, then it may be helpful to consider the following: ask the individual why they are relying on you, discuss this with them and let them know you may not always be available. Relying on one person can promote overdependence, a potential negative where a large focus of care and management in LTCs relates to self-management.
Am I becoming too emotionally involved in this person's care?	If the answer is yes then you need to ask yourself if this is affecting the care you are delivering. (As part of forming therapeutic relationships you invest part of your 'self' in that relationship. Discussing aspects of your personal life may be appropriate if they are used to either help build a relationship or to demonstrate to a person how a situation was managed. However, the focus of that discussion should be the individual and their needs and not be used as an opportunity for you to discuss your needs.)
Is the person and/ or their carer/family viewing me as a member of their family?	If the answer is yes, is this appropriate? (Individuals and/ or carers may promote a friendship with you as this 'normalises' the relationship and allows them to forget the true nature of their relationship with you. This may be part of their coping mechanism and it may be appropriate for you to discuss this with them in order to find other ways in which they can be supported or accept their current situation. This may be especially true for those who are receiving ongoing care in their own homes.)

Table 2.1: Questions to ask yourself to ensure appropriate boundaries are maintained

Meeting the needs of the person

In a therapeutic relationship the needs of the person are assessed at the outset to identify mutually acceptable goals and who is responsible in the achievement of those goals. The needs of the individual are paramount and should be the focus of the relationship. Actively listening to the person, to find out their concerns, worries, etc., reminds us that the therapeutic relationship is there to benefit the person, not the nurse. Asking a simple question such as 'what is the most important thing I can do for you today?' or 'can you tell me why I have been asked to come to see you today?' demonstrates to the individual that your focus is on them and their needs, rather than your interpretation of what their needs might be. This is especially true when caring for those living with an LTC, where one of the main cornerstones of management is self-care: in order to promote self-care and management you must devise a plan of care that clearly reflects the person's needs as this will increase feelings of empowerment and autonomy.

Promoting the autonomy of the person

Autonomy is the freedom to determine one's own actions and behaviours. A relationship where you encourage active involvement of the individual promotes their autonomy and ensures that they are better able to understand their own situation and take active steps to participate in their care. For those living with an LTC, finding out their level of knowledge and understanding about their condition and how much they want to be involved in managing their own care will allow the level of personal autonomy that reflects their wishes. Many people living with an LTC are experts in their care and will possess a great deal of knowledge regarding their care and management. Indeed, it may be you that is asking the person questions about their care and management rather than them asking you.

It must be recognised though that not all individuals will want to be actively involved in their care to the same degree. An elderly gentleman living with Parkinson's disease may take the attitude that managing his condition is the responsibility of the healthcare team: 'that's what they get paid for', whereas a young man living with asthma may actively seek to be more involved in his care: 'I would like to have access to a nebuliser at home and have a clear protocol written that enables me to manage my condition myself should I have an acute asthma attack'. Neither of these approaches is wrong or right, they are just different. By developing a therapeutic relationship you will begin to know what is right for that person and how to ensure a positive experience for that individual.

Ensuring a positive experience for the person

Meeting the needs of those living with an LTC in a caring and sensitive manner will promote a positive experience for the person. This person-centred approach will not only increase their ability to participate in self-care and management but will also assist them in maintaining a more positive outlook in relation to their condition and future.

In order to promote effective therapeutic relationships with individuals living with an LTC it is important to understand the concept of emotional intelligence. Put simply, **emotional intelligence** is about understanding your own emotions and those of others around you. Recognising and developing your own emotional intelligence will impact on the way you deliver care; recognising and developing the emotional intelligence of those living with an LTC has the potential to influence how they live with their condition. We will now look at these aspects of the therapeutic relationship in more detail.

The therapeutic relationship and emotional intelligence

> ### Case study: Frazer
>
> *Frazer is 42 and is living with Type 1 diabetes. In the past he has not always managed his diabetes as effectively as he should. Since the birth of his daughter six years ago, he has taken a more proactive role in managing his diabetes, though he still smokes 10 cigarettes a day. You are working with Frazer's practice nurse today and Frazer is visiting her to have the ulcer on his foot redressed.*
>
> *To ensure that Frazer's care was delivered in a non-judgemental manner you need to have an understanding about how your emotions might impact on the care delivered:*
>
> - *you may feel that Frazer is to blame for his current health issues due to his smoking and previous neglect of his diabetes;*
> - *you may feel that Frazer is being selfish and that he should stop smoking as it is not only damaging his health but also could damage his daughter's health.*
>
> *Frazer's own emotions may also be impacting on his attitude to his diabetes:*
>
> - *he may feel that as his health is already damaged there is no point in stopping smoking;*
> - *he may not be aware of the impact his choices are having on his family.*
>
> *As you can see from the scenario above there is the potential for our emotions and feelings to impact negatively on our interactions with those in our care. There is also the possibility that a person's emotions can have a negative impact on their condition and how they manage it.*

To understand emotional intelligence as a concept we need to go back to Howard Gardner's 'multiple intelligence' theory (Gardner, 1983) to see the first recognition of emotional intelligence, described by Gardener as intrapersonal intelligence. Intrapersonal intelligence is concerned with your capacity to understand yourself, to recognise and appreciate your emotions and to use this information to regulate your life (Gardner, 1999). Acknowledging Gardner's work on intrapersonal intelligence, Salovey and Mayer (1990) developed emotional intelligence as a concept. In their theory intrapersonal intelligence is seen as being part of emotional intelligence. Salovey and Mayer define emotional intelligence as being:

> *the ability to monitor one's own and* **others***' feelings and emotions, to discriminate among them and to use this information to guide one's thinking and actions.*
>
> (Salovey and Mayer, 1990, page 189 (emphasis added))

As you can see, the difference between intrapersonal intelligence and emotional intelligence is the ability to recognise and respond to *others'* emotions. In 1998 the Consortium for Research on Emotional Intelligence in Organisations (Cherniss, 1998) listed the abilities required for emotional intelligence as: self-awareness, self-regulation, motivation, empathy and social skills (see Table 2.2).

Emotional intelligence abilities	Application to practice
Self-awareness	Being aware of your strengths and weaknesses and looking to managing these. You may feel uncomfortable when dealing with conflict and recognise that dealing with conflict is not one of your strengths. The important thing is to act on this and to put strategies in place to address this; one might be to attend an assertiveness course.
Self-regulation	Being aware of your 'self' and your emotions and being able to regulate these and not become overwhelmed by them. When faced with conflict your first response might be to become angry yourself: recognising this and regulating your emotions will avoid an escalation of the situation. Working on your communication skills and de-escalation techniques would help manage this.
Motivation	Your ability to use self-awareness and self-regulation of your emotions to inspire yourself and others. Recognising that you find dealing with conflict challenging and having the desire to improve your ability to manage conflict will motivate you to undertake activities that will increase your skills in this area.
Empathy	Your capacity to understand another's situation, to identify with their emotions and to use this to respond in an appropriate manner. By increasing your knowledge and skills in relation to conflict management, and by reflecting on these, you will increase your ability to empathise with and respond appropriately to individuals/relatives/carers that may be angry.
Social skills	Your capability to influence and to maintain and improve interpersonal relationships through the use of effective and supportive communication skills. Through reflecting on your experience of conflict management and through undertaking assertiveness training you have increased your range of communication skills and are able to use these in other situations to support those in your care.

Table 2.2: Emotional intelligence abilities and their relation to nursing practice

As you can see from Table 2.2, emotional intelligence influences many aspects of nursing care. The utilisation and development of emotional intelligence in relation to you and those in your care will impact on the therapeutic relationship and the delivery of care. Jean (now Baroness) McFarlane, a prominent nurse academic, in 1976 maintained that nursing and caring have similar roots, stating that:

> *caring signifies a feeling of concern: of interest… with a view to protection. Nursing means… to nourish and cherish.*

> (Smith, 1992, page 9)

Your ability to form an emotional connection and to hold a person in unconditional positive regard or **prizing**, will promote their dignity and uniqueness and will ensure that all your interactions have the individual's best interests at the core (Rogers, 1967), enabling you to provide holistic person-centred care.

Activity 2.1   *Reflection*

Case study: Frazer (see website: www.learningmatters.co.uk/nursing for full case scenario)

Reflecting back on the case study mentioned earlier in the chapter how could you demonstrate prizing as it relates to Frazer?

A brief outline answer is given at the end of the chapter.

This ability to *prize* within nursing was the focus of Pam Smith, in her study: *The Emotional Labour of Nursing: How Nurses Care* (Smith, 1992). Smith found that nurses defined themselves by their ability to care, though in order to protect themselves they must possess the knowledge about how to manage their feelings, a pre-requisite for emotional intelligence which is still relevant to nursing today. More recent publications have continued to place emotional intelligence as an integral part of nursing; Freshwater and Stickley (2004) describe emotional intelligence as 'the heart of the art' in nursing, implying that the utilisation of emotional intelligence guides all that nurses do. This application of emotional intelligence to nursing practice supports the notion of caring that only takes place through the development of a person-centred therapeutic relationship. To support you in the development of your 'heart of the art', take the time to undertake Activity 2.2.

Activity 2.2   *Reflection*

As a student nurse you may find yourself in situations that are emotionally challenging; for example, the death of a young child or being faced with an angry relative. It is important that if you are in a situation like this you recognise your limitations, seek support and plan how you will address your limitations. Using the components of emotional intelligence as listed in Table 2.2, identify your strengths and weaknesses in relation to these. Use the following questions as prompts.

- If you are feeling overwhelmed by your emotions, what strategies do you use to manage this?

continued opposite…

---

continued...

- How do you motivate yourself? What strategies do you use to motivate others?
- How do you demonstrate empathy?
- What communication skills do you use when engaging with people?

Once you have identified your strengths and weaknesses compile a personal and professional development plan to address these.

To support you in this task there are many online emotional intelligence tests you can undertake, for example: **http://psychology.about.com/library/quiz/bl_eq_ qu.htm**.

As the answers will be based on your own observations there is no outline answer at the end of this chapter.

Emotional intelligence and understanding those living with an LTC

While Activity 2.2 relates to you and your emotional intelligence it is also important to be aware of emotional intelligence as it relates to individuals living with an LTC. Being diagnosed with an LTC can result in a variety of emotional responses: anger, confusion, loss and despair. It is not only the initial diagnosis that has an emotional impact: living with and managing their condition can also have an emotional impact, and increased stress impacts negatively on both a person's ability to engage in the management of their condition and their self-esteem (McKenna, 2007). A review of available literature by Telford et al. (2005) concluded that for those living with an LTC, displaying appropriate emotional responses and maintaining a positive attitude were shown to influence how effectively they engage in health promotion activities and how well they cope with difficult situations, for example, a deterioration in their condition, and how they manage the resulting stress of this. This is particularly relevant to individuals whose LTC is known to be exacerbated by stress, e.g. systemic lupus erythematosus and rheumatoid arthritis. For example, McKenna (2007) suggests that supporting individuals to increase their self-awareness by supporting them to identify, express and manage their feelings will increase their ability to manage stress and anxiety. Some strategies that could be used to facilitate this are:

- developing their communication skills, e.g. rehearsing important conversations – breaking bad news to their family, assertiveness skills to ensure that they maximise any consultations they have;
- diary keeping and review, e.g. what was good about today, what was not so good, what made this a good day.

Using these strategies and by involving other members of the multidisciplinary team will assist those living with an LTC to emotionally adjust and manage their condition (see the Further reading list at the end of this chapter for additional resources).

The therapeutic relationship and carers

There are approximately six million carers in the UK involved in the direct care of family, friends and partners (Carers UK, 2009). The shift towards community-based care, with the emphasis on maintaining people to live in their own homes for as long as possible, has resulted in a change in the provision of this care, with some aspects of care being delivered by informal carers. Carers play a pivotal role in the care and management of those living with an LTC and can be involved in personal care, such as bathing, dressing and toileting, providing physical health e.g. getting in and out of bed, walking and getting up and down stairs, and administering medication (Carers UK, 2006). The Carers (Equal Opportunities) Act 2004 gives carers the right to an individual assessment of their needs, and must ensure that work, lifelong learning and leisure are considered when a carer is assessed. It should be noted that the Carers Act (2004) only applies to England and Wales; in Scotland it is the *Community Care and Health (Scotland) Act* (2002) that gives carers the right to an individual assessment, and in Northern Ireland the 2006 publication *Caring for Carers: recognising, valuing and supporting the caring role* focuses on the needs of the carer. Yet despite this, Bee et al. (2008) found that there was a consistent lack of practical support available, predominately related to lack of information. While the focus of this review was on end-of-life care in those with cancer, the underlying principles are transferable to those caring for people living with an LTC. Indeed Caress et al. (2008), whose review focused on chronic obstructive pulmonary disease, noted that few of the studies reviewed addressed carers' needs for information and support, with no studies being identified that focused on strategies to enhance the capacity of carers to deliver effective care.

What is the role of the therapeutic relationship between you and the carer in the management of those living with an LTC? When engaging in a therapeutic relationship with a carer, the same principles that you use when engaging with any individual apply, and some of the needs will be the same. It is recognised, however, that carers have specific needs. These include the need for information and support to undertake nursing-based activities (Bee et al., 2008), and the development of coping strategies and ongoing support that recognise the difficulty of caring for someone living with an LTC (Chambers et al., 2001, Carmichael and Hulme, 2008). The focus of the therapeutic relationship between you and the carer must then address these topics, and any others identified, in relation to the needs of the individual carer and their circumstances. Let us now look at these areas and some strategies available to you to support carers.

Information and support to undertake nursing-based activities

It is known that carers undertake nursing-based activities when caring for people living with an LTC (Bee et al., 2008). Providing carers with adequate education and information regarding nursing activities relevant to them will not only enhance the care delivered but will increase carer confidence. Depending on the situation information, advice and education may be required on the following; these themes were identified in Bee et al.'s (2008) review.

- Medication and pain management – education regarding awareness and understanding of the medication being taken including side-effects, how and when it should be taken, understanding of assessment and management of pain.
- Personal hygiene – education and advice regarding skin observation and assessment and use of pressure-relieving aids, management of continence and bathing and use of technical equipment such as hoists.

- Nutrition – information regarding a healthy diet and specific dietary requirements.
- Management of symptoms – information and advice regarding fatigue, weakness and awareness of a person's mental health status.
- Emergency situations – education and advice regarding recognising the signs of an emergency, e.g. myocardial infarction, and who to contact.

As part of The Carers (Recognition and Services) Act 1995, The Carers and Disabled Children Act 2000 and The Carers (Equal Opportunities) Act 2004, carers have the right to have an assessment of their needs made. A carer's assessment gives carers the opportunity to discuss with social services what help they require to enable them to continue caring. Carer assessments are carried out by the local social services department, though a referral to social services for this may come from another healthcare professional, e.g. district nurse. The assessment provides a baseline assessment of how the carer is coping and what they perceive their needs to be in relation to the following.

1. Any aspect of caring: tasks involved in caring, how is your relationship with the person you are caring for and what practical help do you need?

2. The health and wellbeing of the carer: how is your health, do you have any other pressures, e.g. young children, and do you have any free time?

This assessment needs to be handled sensitively, with the carer being aware that the information supplied will be used to provide support for them and ultimately the person they are caring for. Therefore it may be necessary for information to be shared with other members of the health and social care team. For example if the carer is requesting specific support regarding a nursing intervention then you, along with a community nurse, may provide the relevant support. Other practical support offered may be advising about benefits that may be available, providing information about local support groups, and having access to **respite care** services. Further information regarding carer assessment is available via the following website: **www.carersuk. org/Information/Helpwithcaring**.

Children who are carers also have the right of an assessment under the provision of the government acts, e.g. in England it is the Children Act 1989 and The Carers (Equal Opportunities) Act 2004 and in Scotland the Community Care and Health Act (Scotland) 2002. Whichever Act is used to assess a child and their needs as a carer, the focus of the assessment is the same: to find out the amount and level of care being delivered by the child and the impact this has on their leisure and school life. It should be recognised that caring as a child can have significant impact on both the physical and mental health of the child and can impact on their choices and future life achievements. As part of the child assessment it may also be relevant to find out from the parent they are caring for the impact their condition is having, e.g. how does your condition affect your children and how can we support you in your role as a parent?

It is recognised that you may not be directly involved in undertaking a carer assessment. However, increasing your knowledge and having an awareness of the availability of carer assessments will assist you to be responsive to the needs of carers.

Coping and support

Some degree of stress can be productive; indeed stress can increase our motivation to undertake activities, e.g. as a student nurse a stress response to a forthcoming examination may be to plan and undertake a programme of revision. However, it should be noted that too much stress can have a negative impact on our ability to cope. How well the carer is coping with their role should not be ignored – carer stress can have a negative impact on the carer's ability to continue in the caring role (Douglas-Dunbar and Gardiner, 2007). Stress can affect a carer both psychologically and physically: psychologically it can affect their ability to deliver care sensitively and responsively and physically it can determine their ability to safely provide care, especially that requiring physical interventions, e.g. bathing. Carer stress is a possibility for any carer; however, those caring for individuals with a mental health condition, e.g. dementia, may be particularly vulnerable, with specific information and advice being required in relation to understanding and managing challenging behaviours (Papastavrou et al., 2007).

As a nurse it is your responsibility to have an awareness of the role stress and caring have in the provision of care for those living with an LTC. In your role as a nurse you can help carers manage stress by providing them with information about organisations who can help them to manage stress. At the time of writing, Caring with Confidence and Looking after Me are two strategies that support carers living in England. Caring with Confidence is a free programme for carers, established by the Department of Health, that provides carers with information regarding the many aspects of caring, e.g. the emotional aspect of caring for someone and the essentials of caring, i.e., medication. The course is delivered either through the use of local group sessions or online sessions (DH, 2009) and is supported by an easy-to-access website (**www.caringwithconfidence.net/**). Looking after Me is a programme that is part of the Expert Patients Programme and is a free programme that, like Caring with Confidence, focuses on the carer and their needs and addresses topics such as relaxation, healthy eating and planning for the future (Expert Patients Programme, 2009). In Scotland, Wales and Ireland carer support and training is coordinated by the regional organisations of the umbrella organisation Carers UK (**www.carersuk.org/Home**).

Given the demographics of carers, it is likely that a percentage of carers, especially younger ones, will be working. The Employment Act of 2002, which gave employees who care for children under six (18 if the child has special needs) the right to request flexible working, was updated by the government in 2007 to include employees who care for adults. While it is recognised that the act provides employees the right to request flexible working, their request does not have to be granted, with employers having the right to refuse if there is a clear business need that prevents flexible working. At the time of writing, in order to support carers who are not working, financial support is available in the form of the Carer's Allowance. Information regarding the Carer's Allowance can be found at **www.direct.gov.uk/en/caringforsomeone/ moneymatters/dg_10012522**. Research by Carmichael and Hulme in 2008 identified the complexities of financial support for carers, especially in relation to the working/benefits paradox, where carers either felt they had to work as benefits were insufficient or they did not work as this would affect the benefits received.

Activity 2.3 — *Decision-making*

Case study: Angela

Following the initial joy at the birth of his son Charlie and the shock news of Angela's diagnosis of multiple sclerosis, James is struggling to come to terms with his new roles as father and carer.

You are on a primary care placement, and spending the day with the health visitor. Today, you are visiting Angela, James and Charlie to discuss Charlie's progress and to see how the family are managing. When you arrive, Angela is upstairs sleeping, and during your conversation with James it is evident that he is finding it hard to accept Angela's diagnosis and he starts to ask questions about the future and his role.

As part of the team involved in caring for this family, how might you ensure James's needs were assessed and what strategies would you put in place to support him?

A brief outline answer is given at the end of the chapter.

As you can see from Activity 2.3 the carer's role will change over time. Most people do not set out to become carers but rather over a period of time find themselves in that role. It can happen slowly over the course of months or years, due to a gradual deterioration in health, e.g. as a result of heart disease or Parkinson's disease, or it can happen suddenly due to an acute deterioration in health, e.g. as a result of a cerebrovascular accident or other rapidly developing neurological condition. Often the assumption is made that carers are, as they are there and already involved, happy to undertake this role. Developing a therapeutic relationship with carers will enable you to address their changing needs, allowing them to continue in their role as a carer for as long as they wish to do so.

As discussed above it is important that a person-focused therapeutic relationship is in place if you are to provide effective support both to someone living with an LTC and their carer. In order to allow this to happen there has to be an open and honest exchange of information, ideas and wishes. This interactive process echoes that of the therapeutic relationship, and helps to define the need for clear person-centred care and management.

Communication strategies in LTCs

In your role as a nurse caring for those living with an LTC you may be involved in their care at different stages in their journey. This may take the form of helping to understand their diagnosis, providing them with information during an exacerbation of their condition and caring for them during the end stages of their illness. The questions asked by individuals and the nature of the information given at different stages on a person's journey changes. The aim of this section is to focus on specific aspects of communication that relate to caring for people living with an LTC. To support you in the development of more general knowledge and skills regarding your communication there are many other books available, e.g. *Communication and Interpersonal Skills for Nurses* (Bach and Grant, 2009). When caring for people with an LTC it is important to recognise what some of the barriers to communication may be; see box overleaf.

Barriers to communication

For some of those living with an LTC and for those caring for them there are potential barriers to communication that impact on their ability to communicate and to form an effective therapeutic relationship. This can take the form of sensory impairment, e.g. reduction in hearing and/or vision. Some simple strategies to improve communication in this situation are: ensure hearing aids have batteries and glasses are clean, and to access support and equipment through either the Royal National Institute for Deaf People (RNID) or the Royal National Institute of Blind People (RNIB). For those living with a neurological disorder, e.g. Parkinson's disease or cerebrovascular accident, their ability to use non-verbal means of communication, facial expressions and gestures may be limited. Language difficulties, e.g. where English is not the person's or carer's first language, accessing an interpreter service rather than using a family member to interpret is preferable in this situation, especially where sensitive information may be discussed. As a nurse you may also be your own barrier to communication: in challenging situations we may choose to 'close the patient down', enabling us to retain some sense of control, we may change the topic, get into small talk, ignore the question or give false or premature reassurance (Maguire et al., 1996).

Being aware of these barriers, utilising the therapeutic relationship and developing your EI will help minimise these barriers.

Due to the ongoing nature of their condition and the focus on NHS policy to promote self-management it is important that those living with an LTC are enabled to actively take part in the discussions regarding their treatment and management. To facilitate this you can encourage them to use the steps outlined below in the acronym PART to do this; for example, before they attend a consultation with a doctor.

- **P**repare – identify main concerns, prioritise these, and write these down before the consultation. Try to be open in sharing thoughts and feelings, be prepared to concisely describe symptoms, time frame etc., and bring along a list of any medication.
- **A**sk – ask questions about diagnosis and prognosis, tests, treatments and any follow-up; ensure you get the answers you understand.
- **R**epeat – repeat key points in the consultation, to verify your understanding and ensure consultation has been understood; this also allows the doctor to check your understanding.
- **T**ake action – make sure you understand what is going to happen next, ask for instructions to be written down: if the advice being given is not going to be easy to follow then let the doctor know why to see if an alternative can be given.

Activity 2.4   *Communication*

Case study: Andrew

Andrew has COPD and has recently been in hospital due to a chest infection, his second in the last four months. Following each infection his degree of breathlessness has increased.

continued opposite...

continued...

He is due to attend an out-patient appointment next week, and he is concerned about these recent chest infections.

You are on a primary care placement and are visiting Andrew with your mentor, who is Andrew's district nurse. During your visit Andrew begins to express concerns about his forthcoming consultation. How could you use the acronym PART to ensure that Andrew maximises his consultation?

A brief outline answer is given at the end of the chapter.

As you can see from Activity 2.4 it is important to listen to the person to understand their perspective and their needs: in understanding their perspective, you will be able to deliver person-centred care. Actively listening to the individual is a key aspect of this: Epictetus (Greek philosopher, AD 55–c.135) said:

We have two ears and one mouth so that we listen twice as much as we speak.

Your listening skills can be improved by asking open-ended questions: open-ended questions encourage the person to give details and prompt you to follow these up. Use paraphrasing, which involves reflecting back to the person a summary of what they had been saying. Paraphrasing allows you to verify the accuracy of your listening, and accurately demonstrates that you have been listening. Listen first and advise second: if an individual comes to you with a problem you may be tempted to provide a solution; however, allowing the person to talk may allow them to find their own solution. Finally commit completely, remove distractions and focus on the person as this will signal to the person that they are your priority (Boyd, 1998). An effective strategy that can be used in the care of those living with an LTC is narrative-based care.

Narrative-based care: a communication strategy for LTCs

Story-telling can be viewed as a 'children's activity', yet it is through the use of stories that we understand, experience, communicate and create ourselves. Our stories, like our lives, are constantly changing; they consist of the process of telling the story as well as the end product – the story itself. The idea of narrative-based medicine contrasts with that of the medical model, where assessment of the person focuses on signs and on gathering a diagnosis. In narrative-based medicine the focus is on the person and uses their narrative to understand the importance of the illness from their perspective (Launer, 2006). Some narratives may focus on a specific aspect of a person's care and management, e.g. during a consultation with a GP. Alternatively, the narrative may address many aspects of a person's life, e.g. during an initial meeting with a Macmillan nurse. Regardless of the setting narratives should contain characters and setting (who, what and where), plot (sequence of events) and voice or point of view (Launer, 2002). Narratives should be written in collaboration with the person telling the story: it may be that you are required to provide some structure to allow this to happen, and some questions that can be used to assist individuals to provide a narrative are as follows:

- Can you give me an example of when your problem/concern/symptom affected your life?'
- Describe the incident in terms of place, time, and others involved.

- Does this problem affect others, and if so, how?
- What were the sequence of events?
- What did this mean to you at the time, and what does it mean to you now?

Recognising the emotional impact that a diagnosis of an LTC has and providing the person with ways to manage this has a positive psychological effect on their ability to manage their condition. The use of the person's story also places the emphasis of the relationship on them and their needs. Narrative-based medicine has been pioneered in the UK by Greenhalgh and Hurwitz, who in 1999 published in the *British Medical Journal* their article *Narrative-based medicine: why study narrative?* This article focused on a person-centred narrative providing meaning, context and perspective to their situation and it defines how, why and in what way the person is seeking support.

Activity 2.5   *Reflection*

Elsie is a 77-year-old retired school teacher who is recovering from a cerebrovascular accident (CVA) that has resulted in a right hemiplegia and expressive dysphasia. Working with her speech and language therapist she wrote this narrative while in hospital. How would you have used Elsie's narrative to assist you in planning her care?

> No-one really sees me as they walk past. They see the shell of the person I was. This is the first time I have been in hospital and I do not want to be here, if I could talk I would tell them that but I can't. The stroke I had has robbed me of the ability to communicate with the outside world. My stroke has also paralysed my right arm and leg. The doctors do not speak to me but to the nurses – just because I can't speak does not mean that I can't hear. They say I may never walk again – I am not interested in that, I can accept using a wheelchair, after all a wheelchair would allow me more freedom, I could move myself from room to room and decide where I wanted to sit.
>
> I have no-one to come and visit me – you see I never married and my friends, well they are old too and the journey to the hospital is long and tiring. My next of kin is my solicitor. The only visitor I have had is the social worker, Meg. It cannot be easy for her trying to help me when I cannot talk to her, I do try and occasionally I can get a couple of words out, however the harder I concentrate the less I can say. Meg talks to me about going into a nursing home – where I can be looked after. I do not want to be looked after. I want to live independently in my own home. Yet I cannot tell her this, I get frustrated; knock my glass over, start to cry and Meg leaves.
>
> Today the speech therapist came to visit me. Her name is Karen and she took me to a quiet place away from the ward. I spent over an hour with her and she is coming back to see me tomorrow. Karen says it is likely that I will get my speech back though I will always have some difficulty expressing myself. She says her tests show that I have expressive dysphasia, meaning I understand everything I hear but I am unable to find the right words when I talk. Karen has given me a sheet of exercises to do; she says I am to do them three times a day though I am going to aim for five – on waking, after each meal and before I go to bed. At last a glimmer of hope.

As the answers will be based on your own observations there is no outline answer at the end of this chapter.

As you can see from Activity 2.5 it may not always be possible to obtain a narrative of events from a person in your care, for example those with sensory impairments or dementia. Working with carers and family members to build up a narrative will demonstrate effective use of your emotional intelligence as the use of narrative encourages empathy and promotes understanding of the person and their needs. It may supply us with useful clues that can contribute to a holistic assessment of those in our care, allowing us to set a person-centred agenda.

Conclusion

Having read this chapter and worked through the activities you will have developed your knowledge and skills in relation to the therapeutic relationship and long term conditions. How you use these will depend on where you are working and your roles and responsibilities. However, as a nurse you can improve communication with those in your care and their family/carer in many ways. By increasing your level of emotional intelligence you can be yourself, be open and honest, recognise and acknowledge your limitations and take personal responsibility. By engaging in a therapeutic relationship with individuals and/or their carers you can work as part of a team by listening and responding to their needs. By using communication strategies like narrative-based care you can increase the wellbeing of the person/carer, improve physical and mental state, promote a better adjustment to illness and increase an individual's sense of control (Wallace, 2001).

Chapter summary

This chapter has provided you with an overview of the role of the therapeutic relationship in relation to LTC; it has also outlined the importance of emotional intelligence as a factor in the therapeutic relationship, both for you and for those in your care. This has emphasised the importance of person-focused care in the delivery of care for those living with an LTC as this is a key message in recent health policy. It has focused on the importance of recognising the role of carers and working with them to support both carers and those living with an LTC. Some specific communication strategies useful in the care and management of LTCs have been discussed and related to clinical practice.

Activities: brief outline answers

Activity 2.1: Reflection (page 36)

You could demonstrate prizing with Frazer through the use of both verbal and non-verbal communication skills, some of which might be:

- verbal: encouraging interaction by asking open questions, using non-judgemental language and demonstrating active listening by reflecting back to Frazer what he has been saying;
- non-verbal: by making and maintaining eye contact, using open gestures, using gestures that will encourage Frazer to talk, e.g. smiling, nodding and by spending time with Frazer.

Using these skills would demonstrate you were actively listening to him and valuing and respecting what he was saying. However, to be able to 'prize' Frazer fully it may also be necessary for you to recognise and overcome any prejudices you may have regarding how Frazer has managed his condition in the past. Doing with will ensure that any communication you have is not subconsciously affected by your emotions.

Activity 2.3: Decision-making (page 41)

By involving a social worker in this family's care you could ask that a carer assessment be carried out, allowing social support and financial support to be offered. From a nursing perspective it may be appropriate to establish how much knowledge and understanding James has in relation to multiple sclerosis, e.g. likely disease progression, prognosis etc. It may also be appropriate to provide information about accessing support groups and/or carer training courses; it may also be worth suggesting to James that Angela attends an Expert Patients Programme if she has not done so. You would need to ensure that this information was delivered in a sensitive and timely manner; you would not want to overwhelm James with information. It would also be important to ensure that any information given had been understood – this could be reviewed at a follow-up visit.

Activity 2.4: Communication (page 42)

To help Andrew prepare for his consultation you could assist him to identify his main concerns and to write these down. These may relate to his recent chest infections or to his increasing breathlessness. Encourage Andrew to share how he is feeling – is his increasing breathlessness beginning to affect his mood? Find out from Andrew if he has any specific questions that he would like answered – do the recurring chest infections mean his disease is getting worse? Help Andrew to write down his questions, and remind him to take some paper and a pen with him so he can write down the answers. Remind Andrew that this is his consultation and that before he leaves he should review with his consultant what has been said.

Further reading

Bach, S and Grant A (2011) *Communication and Interpersonal Skills for Nurses*, 2nd edn. Exeter: Learning Matters
A useful introduction for nursing students to the complexities of communication skills.

Bayliss, J (2001) *Counselling Skills in Palliative Care*. Wiltshire: Quay books.
While addressing communication in palliative care, many aspects can be transferred to those living with an LTC.

Chilton, S, Melling, K, Drew, D and Clarridge, A (2004) *Nursing in the Community: An Essential Guide to Practice*. London: Hodder Arnold.
Provides a comprehensive overview of all aspects of community nursing. Chapter 5 focuses on therapeutic relationships.

McKenna, J (2007) Emotional intelligence training in adjustment to physical disability and illness. *International Journal of Therapy and Rehabilitation*.14 (12), 551–56.
This article discusses emotional intelligence and how it can be used to help people adjust to disability or illness.

Useful websites

www.carersuk.org/Home
Provides a gateway to all carer UK sites, e.g. Scotland, Northern Ireland and Wales; offers advice and information for carers.

Chapter 3
Health promotion in long term conditions

NMC Standards for Pre-registration Nursing Education

This chapter will address the following competencies:

Domain 1: Professional values

3. All nurses must support and promote the health, wellbeing, rights and dignity of people, groups, communities and populations. These include people whose lives are affected by ill-health, disability, ageing, death and dying. Nurses must understand how these activities influence public health.
4. All nurses must work in partnership with service users, carers, families, groups, communities and organisations. They must manage risk, and promote health and wellbeing while aiming to empower choices that promote self-care and safety.

Domain 2: Communication and interpersonal skills

6. All nurses must take every opportunity to encourage health promoting behaviour through education, role modelling and effective communication.

Domain 3: Nursing practice and decision-making

8. All nurses must provide educational support, facilitation skills and therapeutic nursing interventions to optimise health and wellbeing. They must promote self-care and management whenever possible, helping people to make choices about their healthcare needs, involving families and carers where appropriate, to maximise their ability to care for themselves.

NMC Essential Skills Clusters

This chapter will address the following ESCs:

Cluster: Care, compassion and communication

2. People can trust the newly registered graduate nurse to engage in person-centred care empowering people to make choices about how their needs are met when they are unable to meet them themselves.

By the second progression point:

2. Actively empowers people to be involved in the assessment and care planning process.

By entry to the register:

8. is sensitive and empowers people to meet their own needs and make choices and considers the person and their carer(s) and their capability to care.

continued overleaf...

• • *continued...* •

Cluster: Organisational aspects of care

9. People can trust the newly registered graduate nurse to treat them as partners and work with them to make a holistic and systematic assessment of their needs; to develop a personalised plan that is based on mutual understanding and respect for their individual situation promoting health and wellbeing, minimising risk of harm and promoting their safety at all times.

By the second progression point:

3. Understands the concept of public health and the benefits of healthy lifestyles and the potential risks involved with various lifestyles or behaviours, for example, substance misuse, smoking, obesity.

4. Recognises indicators of unhealthy lifestyles.

By entry to the register:

16. Promotes health and wellbeing, self-care and independence by teaching and empowering people and carers to make choices in coping with the effects of treatment and the ongoing nature and likely consequences of a condition including death and dying.

Chapter aims

After reading this chapter you will be able to:

* explain the importance of health promotion for people living with an LTC;
* understand the influence of health determinants in the care and management of people living with an LTC;
* identify, describe and apply approaches to health promotion in the care and management of LTCs;
* understand and describe the process of motivational interviewing and its role in the care and management of LTCs.

Introduction

Low cost, simple approaches are the key to saving 35 million lives globally by 2015
(Dr Robert Beaglehole, Director Chronic Diseases and Health Promotion, WHO)

Health promotion is a key strategy for use in the care and management of people living with an LTC. The Ottowa Charter for Health Promotion states that the aim of health promotion is to enable people to increase the level of control they have over their health. Increasing a person's ability to positively influence and affect their health can have a positive impact on their quality of life, by addressing not just physical but mental and social wellbeing (WHO, 2009). In order to successfully engage a person with an LTC in health-promoting behaviour it is important that you know and understand them and their lives. Using the therapeutic relationship, as discussed in Chapter 2, as your means of providing person-centred communication and care will contribute to your delivery of health promotion. Increasing a person's ability to positively influence and affect their health not only has a positive impact on their quality of life but also could save their life. It should also be recognised that for many carers the act of caring for a person with an LTC can impact negatively on their health, therefore engaging them in health promotion, if required, will support them in the role as a carer. See Chapter 2 for information on supporting carers and improving their health and wellbeing.

Activity 3.1   *Reflection*

Thinking back to your clinical experience and your role as a health promoter, answer the following questions.

- What health promotion have you been involved in that related to a person living with an LTC?
- How did you carry out your health promotion?
- How did you evaluate the effectiveness of your health promotion?

If you have not been involved in any health promotion intervention then reflect on the health promotion you have seen your mentor involved in.

As the answer will be based on your own observations there is no outline answer at the end of the chapter.

Activity 3.1 reminds you about the health promotion interventions you have been involved in with people in your care who are living with an LTC. This might include, for example, the importance of wearing compression stockings and doing daily active limb exercises following hip replacement surgery for a person living with osteoarthritis. These interventions encourage people to learn about their condition, understand the importance of self-care and then to actively participate and be involved in their care. This approach empowers the person, increasing their sense of control over their situation. If we look at the example above it also minimises the risk of post operative complications, e.g. deep vein thrombosis, therefore reducing the person's length of stay in hospital. In order for your intervention to be a success it is important that you understand about empowerment, health promotion approaches and their use and how to evaluate your intervention. It is important to understand, however, that health promotion should not just be about an individual's health and wellbeing. It should target whole populations and communities. The health promotion intervention mentioned previously may positively impact on the person's health while they are in your care. However, the long term benefits of this health promotion intervention are affected, on discharge home, by the person's family, social support and network and their local environment.

This example not only highlights the integral part that health promotion plays in your day-to-day activity as a nurse but also of the importance aspects such as the environment have on a person's health. This is especially true for people living with an LTC and their carers, where lack of general fitness, mobility or time makes access to services even more difficult. To support you in your ability to promote health in people living with an LTC, this chapter aims to develop your knowledge and understanding of health promotion in relation to the care and management of LTCs. To do this the chapter will focus on developing your knowledge, skills and attributes in relation to health promotion approaches and how to use these to empower people with an LTC to manage their own health condition. Firstly though, to enable you to better support people living with an LTC, this chapter will discuss the factors that contribute to a person's overall health and wellbeing (Naidoo and Wills, 2009) and the influence they have on a person's health, and how **public health** can minimise these.

Policy review

Health promotion and empowerment within the care and management of people living with an LTC has become one of the key priorities, across the UK, with all countries publishing relevant policy documents. In England, health promotion was integral to the National Service Frameworks published by the DH, including coronary heart disease, mental health and older people. More recently in England an important document was *Your health, your way – a guide to long term conditions and self care* (DH, 2009). This publication focuses on enabling people living with an LTC to become more involved in their care and management, with an aspect of this being in relation to adopting healthy lifestyle choices. In Scotland the government published *Long Term Conditions Collaborative: high impact changes* (The Scottish Government Health Delivery Directorate Improvement Support Team, 2009). High impact changes 2 and 3 emphasised the need for self-management for people living with an LTC, with elements of this relating to lifestyle choices and adaptation. The Long Term Conditions Alliance Northern Ireland (2008) again emphasised the importance of health and wellbeing with people living with an LTC having a key role in managing their health and staying healthy. The stated challenge in Wales is *to improve health and wellbeing and reduce the incidence and impact of chronic conditions.* This is seen as being achieved through adopting healthy lifestyles, improving the quality of life for people living with an LTC and increasing independence. Within the care and management of LTCs, health promotion means working with the person concerned to find out what their health issues are and collaborating with them to find ways of empowering them to promote and maintain their own health.

The influence of health when living with an LTC

As discussed in Chapter 1 the majority of care and management you will be involved in when supporting people living with an LTC takes place in primary care. It may be that, during an acute episode or deterioration in their condition, a person is admitted to secondary care where you are involved in delivering specific care and management. However, on a day-to-day basis people living with an LTC manage their condition either independently or with support from you as part of their primary healthcare team. Their care and management take place in their own home, they live their life in their local community and contribute to the local area. It is important therefore that you have an understanding of how their 'life' (behavioural, social, economic, emotional and spiritual) can influence and affect their LTC and their overall sense of health.

Determinants of health

There are many factors that affect the health of a person and their community, and it is these factors that are called determinants of health and can determine how healthy a person is at the present and may be in the future. The health of a person depends on many factors that influence and impact on their life, e.g. genetics, education, environment (WHO, 2010). Table 3.1 discusses the determinants of health and their relevance to your nursing practice.

Determinants of health	Relevance to practice
Genetic and biological factors	Genetics can play a large part in determining a person's lifespan and general health, e.g. Huntington's disease is caused by a faulty gene on chromosome 4, and this faulty gene leads to nerve cell damage in the basal ganglia and cerebral cortex, resulting in uncontrolled muscular movement and cognitive impairment. A person born to a parent with Huntington's disease has a 50:50 chance of inheriting the faulty gene and developing the disease. This is, therefore, a determinant of health that a person can do nothing about; any intervention to manage this depends on advances in medical science. However, genetic counselling can be useful in assisting the family to understand the risks family members experience and how these can be managed.
A person's characteristics and behaviours	How a person adapts and manages stress and challenges in their life can influence their health. Those with reduced coping abilities are more likely to experience negative health and may be less willing to access services (Telford et al., 2005). It is important to recognise this when supporting those with mental health disorders, when supporting those who are recently bereaved or have experienced some other traumatic event. Developing a person's coping mechanisms can increase their sense of empowerment and can positively impact on this aspect of their health. A person's lifestyle behaviours can determine their health, e.g. smoking has been shown as a causative factor in many lung diseases. Providing the opportunity for health promotion in relation to smoking cessation has the potential to positively impact on this aspect of a person's health.

continued overleaf...

continued...

Determinants of health	Relevance to practice
A person's social and economic environment	Higher education levels, income and social status are linked to better health, with those in the highest social class (bank managers, doctors, teachers) living on average seven years more than those in the lower social classes (cleaners, train drivers). Reducing health inequalities and promoting health for those in the lower social classes are two of the main focuses of public health policy (Marmot Review, 2010). Initiatives implemented throughout the UK, such as Sure Start and Health Action Zones, have promoted the development of partnerships across organisations and have helped improve access to services in disadvantaged areas.
A person's physical environment and social support network	A person's ability to move around their physical environment and to feel part of their local community can influence their health and wellbeing (Walker, 2005): what public services are available and accessible to the local community, e.g. is there a local shop, community centre or what are public transport links like? What support is available from their local community – do they have friends locally? You may be planning a person's discharge post hip replacement; they are mobilising but will be requiring ongoing physiotherapy on discharge. They need to be able to access a pharmacy for their medication – where is this and can the person get to it? More importantly through maybe the person's Tuesday lunch club that she attends – this is her opportunity to meet and socialise, and recognising this as part of her discharge plan will be just as important as accessing pharmacy services.

Table 3.1: Determinants of health and their relevance to practice

Activity 3.2   *Critical thinking*

Case study: Andrew

Andrew is 75 years old, a widower. His wife Elizabeth died 10 years ago, and prior to his retirement Andrew was a painter and decorator. Andrew felt very alone when his wife died; they lived for each other and did not have any children. He lives alone in a one-bedroomed flat in sheltered housing accommodation and likes the company this gives him. Recently their live-in warden retired and she was not replaced. The lack of a live-in warden has worried Andrew – he liked to know she was there should he need her. Andrew has been living with COPD for the past 23 years, and he still smokes – he has tried to stop

continued opposite...

continued...

but has always started smoking again. At the moment Andrew does not have any outside assistance – he is able to manage his own personal hygiene and keep his flat clean, as he says one person doesn't make much mess. He is able to walk to his local shop, though due to his COPD and recurring chest infections this takes him some time and he has to stop to rest. He is reluctant to use public transport to travel to the shops in the centre of town.

How does Andrew's current situation influence, either negatively or positively, the determinants of health listed in Table 3.1?

A brief outline answer is given at the end of the chapter.

As Activity 3.2 demonstrates, determinants of health are personal to individuals and their situation and can have both a negative and positive effect on a person's health. As a result there can be large variations in the health of different groups within the population. For example, a girl born in 2006 in Kensington and Chelsea in London has a life expectancy of 87.8 years, more than ten years higher that in Glasgow City, where her life expectancy would be 77.1 years (Office of National Statistics, 2009). It is these inequalities in health of the population, and how to minimise the impact of them, that is the remit of public health. Public health is a high priority on the health agenda throughout the UK, with each national government's public health strategy focused on reducing health inequalities. Web links to each of these sites can be found at the end of this chapter. Having an understanding of the determinants of health and the role public health has in minimising health equalities will enable you to provide effective health promotion for people living with an LTC.

Health promotion and LTCs

Health promotion is the process of enabling people to increase control over, and to improve, their health. It moves beyond a focus on individual behaviour towards a wide range of social and environmental factors.
(World Health Organization, 2010)

As a nurse caring for people living with an LTC, the health promotion you deliver will focus on improving that person's health whatever the stage of their disease progression. Health promotion will be a part of your care and management from diagnosis right through to the palliative stages of their illness. In the early stages of a diagnosis your health promotion will focus on providing health promotion that will lessen the complications of the condition, e.g. increasing their knowledge of their condition. Later in the progression of the disease the health promotion you deliver will be aimed at restoring their highest level of functioning following an exacerbation, e.g. pulmonary rehabilitation. Finally, in the palliative stages of their illness, the health promotion you engage in will focus on improving their quality of life, e.g. through effective symptom management. While the health promotion may be part of your care and management at different times in a person's health journey, the underlying principles of health promotion remain the same. This process of working together with a person living with an LTC relies on that person being able to understand and to act on the information you provide and use this to maintain and maximise their health. This level of engagement will allow the person to actively participate in the health promotion process, empowering them to take control of their health and wellbeing. The ability of a person to do this is dependent of their level of health literacy, that is, their capability to access, understand and use information to maintain their health (Rowlands, 2009). Low health literacy can have a negative effect on a person's ability to engage in health promotion and ultimately on their health. To address this, in England and Wales, the DH and the Department for Business, Innovation and Skills jointly fund the Skilled for Health Programme (ContinYou, 2010). By embedding language, literacy and numeracy into health improvement topics (e.g. healthy eating), the benefits are two-fold. Participants on the programme gain knowledge and understanding in relation to healthy eating but also improve their level of ability in language, literacy and numeracy. Nutbeam (2000, p264) describes health literacy as follows:

> *Health literacy is more than being able to read pamphlets and make appointments. By improving people's access to health information and their capacity to use it effectively, health literacy is crucial to empowerment.*

It is important therefore that you present health promotion information in a format and manner that is relevant to the person, their level of health literacy and their situation. A person's level of health literacy will also influence what approach you use to deliver the health promotion intervention.

Approaches to health promotion

As Activity 3.1 suggests, health promotion can be approached in a variety of ways and often more than one approach is used. This is particularly relevant for those living with an LTC who may require health promotion to be delivered using more than one approach. For a person living with asthma, health promotion is delivered using the medical model when they access flu vaccination programmes, and the empowerment model is used when supporting them to manage asthma attacks without having to access secondary care. In order to provide health promotion to what can be a complex group of people, and in a way that is meaningful, it is important to have an understanding of these approaches and their relevance in the care and management of people living with an LTC. The focus on health promotion here is in relation to the care and management of LTCs. For other aspects of health promotion, see the Further reading list at the end of this chapter.

Medical approach

The medical approach is aimed at populations or groups of people and endeavours to prevent ill health and premature death. It can take the form of primary prevention – prevention of the onset of disease, e.g. through vaccination programmes. Secondary prevention addresses disease progression through the use of screening, e.g. cervical screening programmes, and tertiary prevention focuses on reducing further disability in those who are already ill, e.g. cardiac rehabilitation programmes. The aim of these interventions is to minimise the risk of the population developing specific conditions and they are based on the **epidemiology** of these diseases. The success of these interventions is dependent on people accessing vaccination programmes and screening and evaluated through the analysis of data, indicating a reduction in disease rates and associated mortality. The medical approach is clearly focused on minimising the impact of disease, of which there have been some successes, including the eradication of small pox through vaccination (Naidoo and Wills, 2009). However, living with an LTC is more complex than this might suggest and the medical model does not necessarily address the role that society and the environment play in promoting a person's health. Though this approach will impact on the health of people living with an LTC, accessing cardiac rehabilitation will maintain and promote a person's health and minimise further complications.

Behaviour approach

As discussed earlier (page 51) it is recognised that a person's behaviours can have either a positive or negative effect on their health. The behaviour change approach attempts to encourage people to adopt healthy behaviours which will then improve their health. This approach believes that people own their health and that people can improve their health by adopting healthy lifestyle choices; it also assumes that if people do not take responsibility for their own health then they are responsible for the consequences. Evaluating whether a behaviour change intervention has been successful is long term; the impact of the behaviour change may only become noticeable in time (Naidoo and Wills, 2009). However, it should be recognised that there are many reasons why people do not engage in healthy lifestyle choices, e.g. lack of information, lack of confidence. These should be acknowledged and should be seen as integral to any health promotion intervention. Many recent health promotion strategies (such as Change4Life) have adopted a behaviour change approach and have been delivered centrally by government. This can lead to the perception that people are being told how to live their lives. However, for people living with an LTC and their carers, behaviour change approaches can be used successfully once particular needs have been identified and the intervention targeted to meet those specific needs.

Educational approach

The intention of the educational approach is to provide people with knowledge and information that will enable them to develop the necessary skills to make informed choices about their health behaviours. Unlike the behaviour change approach the educational approach does not set out to effect a change in a particular direction. Rather, it attempts to increase a person's knowledge so that they will be moved towards an informed change in attitude towards their health behaviour. This, in turn, will lead to a positive change in their health behaviour. Educational health promotion programmes are usually led by a teacher or facilitator, and the issues discussed decided by those on the programme. Evaluation of the educational approach may be difficult; people may have increased knowledge and understanding about their health behaviour but may not make the necessary change (Naidoo and Wills, 2009). An example of this type of health promotion approach is the DAFNE (dose adjustment for normal eating) training course for people living with Type 1 diabetes. This is a structured teaching programme where those participating in the programme share their experiences and practise the skills of carbohydrate estimation and dose adjustment. Providing people living with an LTC, and their carers, with relevant information regarding their condition and how to manage it can increase their sense of control and empowerment.

Empowerment approach

The aim of the empowerment approach is concerned with enabling people to take more control over their health and health behaviours. This approach will not be new to you. As a nurse you empower those in your care through the development of person-centred care plans. It is a 'bottom up' approach with the person identifying their own needs and the 'professional', acting as a facilitator, initiating the process and then allowing the person to find their own solutions by increasing their knowledge and skills. Evaluation of this type of intervention is problematic as it is hard to quantify: it is not reflected in the statistics for disease incidence. It is more likely to be evident in the overall affect of a person and their engagement with their situation (Naidoo and Wills, 2009). An example of this might be the use of reminiscence therapy for people living with dementia. The aim of the intervention is to increase the person's sense of who they are and to enable those involved in their care to see more of the person, allowing for planning and delivery of more person-centred care.

Research summary: Reminiscence therapy

Reminiscence therapy (RT) has been used as a therapeutic intervention in the care and management of people with dementia since the 1980s (Cook, 1984). It involves the sharing of memories and uses materials such as old pictures, songs, objects and newspaper articles to trigger these memories. It is suitable for use with people whose dementia is mild to moderate as they are able to access and share distant memories (Brooker Luce, 2000). There is a growing evidence base in support of RT, but further research is needed. Accessing day hospitals offering care for people with dementia, Brooker and Luce (2000) compared levels of wellbeing in people with mild to moderate dementia. They did this through the use of three activities: RT, group activities (structured craft and games activities) and unstructured time (free time with little involvement of staff). Their results indicated that those participating in RT had a greater level of wellbeing compared with those who had taken part in the group activities and unstructured time. It should also be noted that the group activity had a positive effect on wellbeing though not as much as the RT. Their results suggest that the effectiveness of the RT lies in its ability to enable people with different levels of ability to participate and that using RT prompts a person's full range of senses to be engaged. More recently in Japan (Okumura et al., 2008; Nawate et al., 2008) and Taiwan (Huang et al., 2009) the benefits of RT in people with dementia have been researched. In each study the format of the RT varied: Okumura et al. (2008) focused on themes for each session, e.g. childhood play; Nawate et al. (2008) and Huang et al. (2009) brought together RT and cooking. The results of all three studies demonstrated an increase in participants' cognitive function and overall sense of wellbeing and happiness. Huang et al. (2009) showed an improvement in the communication between the care givers and the person with dementia, resulting in increased social interaction.

Social change approach

This approach accepts the role that the socioeconomic environment plays in determining health, and this reflects the impact that these aspects have in determining a person's overall health as can be seen from Activity 3.2. The social change approach endeavours to promote health through bringing about change in the physical, social and economic environment, and can be summed up in the phrase *to make the healthy choice the easier choice.* This approach requires involvement from many areas from the government down and involves legislation, policy planning and implementation and is evaluated by looking at outcomes such as legislative or regulatory changes (Naidoo and Wills, 2009). As a nurse you may not be directly involved in this approach to health promotion; however, you may, as a result of it, undertake health promotion interventions with individuals. For example, a person with coronary heart disease and who smokes may, due to the legislation that prohibits smoking in public places and the rising cost of cigarettes, decide to stop smoking. She then accesses support via her practice nurse who you are working with. While it may have been changes in legislation that prompted her to stop smoking this will impact positively on her coronary heart disease as well as her pocket.

To enable you to apply the above health promotion approaches to your clinical practice, take the time to undertake Activity 3.3. This will allow you to critically apply the above approaches to a person living with an LTC.

Activity 3.3   *Critical thinking*

Case study: Angela

Following her diagnosis of RRMS, Angela has been experiencing wakeful nights. She manages to get to sleep, but if she wakes in the night she lies awake thinking about her condition and worries about how it might affect her and her family in the future. Her wakeful nights have a knock-on effect during the day; she is tired and has less energy to play with her son Charlie. You are visiting Angela with Charlie's health visitor today and Angela mentions her sleepless nights.

What health promotion approaches would you use, and why, to plan a health promotion intervention to improve Angela's quality of sleep?

To further develop your understanding of health promotion strategies as they relate to people with LTCs you can use the other case studies available on the website **www. learningmatters.co.uk/nursing** to integrate theory to your practice.

A brief outline answer is given at the end of the chapter.

Having undertaken Activity 3.3, you will see that your health promotion intervention was driven by Angela. She is concerned about her sleepless nights, is motivated to make a change and is asking you and her health visitor for some advice and support. By working with Angela to devise strategies to change her behaviour you will enable her to improve her health in the short term and will equip her with the skills to manage her condition in the future.

Motivation and health promotion

Dixon (2008) recognises that the success, or not, of a health promotion intervention can relate to how motivated a person is to participate and, in turn, how committed they are to making the change. It can be seen therefore that a person's motivation to participate in health promotion can influence how successful they are going to be in maintaining their health change. Motivation can either be intrinsic or extrinsic. Intrinsic motivation comes from within: I have a desire to change my behaviour, I am self-motivated and I know the change will improve my health. Extrinsic motivation comes from external influences: I have a desire to change my behaviour because if I stop smoking I will save money. To maximise a person's participation in their health promotion it is important to understand what factors influence their motivation to change – are they extrinsic and/or intrinsic (Dixon, 2008)? One of the more popular models that addresses motivation in relation to health promotion is the transtheoretical approach (DiClemente, 2007): this identifies stages that a person progresses and relapses through while making changes in their health behaviour. People can join at any stage and it is often represented in a cyclical way. Table 3.2 describes the stages of the transtheoretical model and outlines some of the strategies and their aims that may be implemented. To assist you in relating this to your care and management of people living with an LTC the transtheoretical model has been related to Frazer, one of the case studies you are following in this book. See box for further information.

Case study: Frazer

Frazer is 42 and is living with Type 1 diabetes. In the past he has not always managed his diabetes as effectively as he should, this has resulted in peripheral neuropathy. Frazer has an ulcer on his foot that is not healing; he attends the practice nurse regularly to have this redressed. Attempts by his practice nurse to encourage Frazer to stop smoking have failed; he still smokes ten cigarettes a day.

What stage is Frazer at?	Your aim is...	Your strategy is...
Pre-contemplation – here Frazer is not intending to make a change in his health behaviour. He may be unmotivated or resistant to making a change, though he may also be concerned about his health behaviour.	To raise awareness with Frazer of the impact his smoking is having on his health and the health of his family.	To provide Frazer with relevant information in an appropriate format, this may be written, audio or visual. You would then revisit this information with Frazer at follow-up visits.
Contemplation – at this stage Frazer may be stating to you his desire to change his health behaviour by stopping smoking. Frazer may be weighing up the pros and cons of stopping smoking.	To allow Frazer to see the benefits of stopping smoking – both in relation to his health and the health of his family.	To explore the advantages of stopping smoking with Frazer. However, you will need to acknowledge with him some of the disadvantages and challenges he may face.

continued opposite...

continued...

Preparation – here Frazer is stating his intention to change his health behaviour by stopping smoking. Frazer now has to commit to a plan that will enable him to change his health behaviour.	To assist Frazer to manage and overcome any challenges to stopping smoking.	To form a plan of action with Frazer that will enable him to change his behaviour. This may involve providing him with information in relation to nicotine patches and how to manage withdrawal symptoms. Establishing links with a support group would also be beneficial for Frazer.
Action – at this stage Frazer has made a recent change (within six months) to his health behaviour by stopping smoking. At this stage Frazer's new behaviour is established.	To use an effective therapeutic relationship to support Frazer to adapt and maintain his health behaviour change.	To review Frazer's plan of action with him, to provide positive reinforcement of his success to date. To encourage Frazer to maintain contact with support group for ongoing support in the transition from smoker to non-smoker, e.g. recognition of trigger factors for his smoking.
Maintenance – here Frazer has maintained his health behaviour change and is no longer smoking. He has integrated his change into his lifestyle.	To provide ongoing support to Frazer.	To minimise the risk of Frazer relapsing by evaluating his success so far and to plan coping strategies that would limit the risk of a relapse, e.g. relaxation techniques, creating rewards for the new behaviour.

Table 3.2: DiClimente's transtheoretical model (2007) and its relevance to your practice

It should be recognised that the successful behaviour change is not always maintained and that relapses may occur. To minimise this it is important that you ensure that each stage is addressed comprehensively and that the aim identified is supported with appropriate strategies. This will give the person the best opportunity to succeed; however, should they relapse they will have to revisit the stages, paying particular attention to any that were not fully addressed (DiClemente, 2007). The transtheoretical model provides a useful framework for targeting health promotion interventions depending on how ready, or otherwise, Frazer is to change his behaviour. However, it does not provide you with a specific strategy you could use in your health promotion intervention to enable Frazer to make changes. One such strategy is motivational interviewing.

Motivational interviewing: a behaviour change strategy to promote health in people living with an LTC

Motivational interviewing (MI) is a person-centred strategy that, through the use of effective communication skills, helps people to explore how they feel about changing their health behaviours (Mason, 2008). By enabling a person to explore their feelings in relation to their behaviour change and giving them the time to work through these it is likely that their intrinsic motivation to change is going to increase. This is due to the fact that they have reached the decision to change their behaviour themselves and have therefore increased their motivation and self-efficacy. Your role in motivational interviewing is to understand why a person might resist change, to actively listen to them and understand their motivations (what are the pros and cons of changing) and in doing so empower them to make their change. The skills you would use and their application to your practice (Carrier, 2009) are outlined in Table 3.3.

Using the skills opposite will enable you to find out if a person is ready to make a change in their behaviour. If they are ready to make a change then it is useful to find out what changes they feel able to make as this places control with the person. You can help by breaking a major change down into smaller more achievable steps to maintain the person's self-efficacy (Carrier, 2009). The use of MI places the person at the centre of the decisions in relation to changing their behaviour. Through the use of open questions you can encourage them to set the agenda. In sharing information with them, by finding out what they know and then providing relevant information you can encourage them to think about how the information applies to them. This approach encourages person-centred health promotion that acknowledges the role that the person has to play in maintaining a successful behaviour change.

Health promotion and learning disability

It is known that people with learning disabilities (LD) experience the same range of health concerns as the general population. Indeed, many people living with a learning disability are at an increased risk of developing specific LTCs –for example people with Down's syndrome have an increased risk of developing ischaemic heart disease (Royal College of Nursing, 2006). However, people with a learning disability are likely to receive lower levels of health promotion and often rely on their family or carer to identify and communicate their health needs to healthcare professionals (Felce et al., 2008). The approaches and strategies discussed in this chapter are relevant to the promotion of health in this group of people; however, it is important to realise that access to and ability to engage in health promotion may be limited for some people, on account of their learning disability. Understanding the barriers (Lindsey, 2002) that might prevent people with an LD accessing health promotion will help you to plan and deliver appropriate interventions.

- Learning and communication difficulties – a person with an LD may not understand or appreciate the significance of a healthy lifestyle or understand the importance of health

MI skill	How you would use it in your practice
Using open questions	Using open questions encourages a person to explore how they feel about a particular behaviour. For example, rather than asking the question 'do you smoke after each meal?' you could ask 'how do you feel about having a cigarette after each meal?'. This not only allows the person to explore their feelings but also helps you to understand the person and their feelings better.
Active and reflective listening	By actively listening to a person and reflecting back what they have said you can demonstrate that you have understood what the person has said. For example, hearing the statement 'I would like to take more exercise, I have put on some weight over the past few months', and by reflecting back to the person like this: 'you are able to see the connection between your lack of exercise and your weight', you will encourage the person to explore their feelings further.
Rolling with resistance	There will be times during discussions about behaviour change where a person is resistant to what you are saying. In MI it is important that you 'roll with the resistance' and respond in an understanding way. Resistance can be reduced by reassuring a person that they are under no obligation to change: 'I am here to support you to lose weight, I am not going to force you to change'. Resistance can also be reduced by recognising when a person may not be ready to discuss a situation: 'From what you are saying you don't sound ready to talk about this today, shall we discuss this at another meeting?'

Table 3.3: MI skills and their application to your clinical practice

screening. This can result in the person not participating in the health promotion activity or not mentioning when they feel unwell as they may not realise the significance of the symptoms. By providing information in an appropriate format, e.g. picture book, providing people with an LD with the opportunity to learn about their health and working with carers you will improve your delivery of health promotion to this client group. An example of this is a health promotion strategy aimed at enabling people with an LD to learn about personal and sexual health (Knight, 2009). Topics include contraception, checking for testicular cancer and sexually transmitted infections.

- Poor carer and professional awareness – carers themselves may not be aware of the importance of a healthy lifestyle, and healthcare professionals may misinterpret changes as being due to the LD rather than another health need. By working with carers to improve their knowledge and understanding and by maintaining your own personal and professional development, you will enhance both the health of the carer and person with an LD.

- Discrimination – there is the potential for carers and professionals to undervalue people with an LD and to neglect their healthcare needs. Understanding your attitudes and beliefs, and that of society's, towards people with an LD will influence the care you deliver. One health promotion campaign is the Inclusive Fitness Initiative (**www.inclusivefitness.org/index.php**): this is aimed at increasing the accessibility of fitness facilities to people with a disability through staff training, developing accessible and inclusive environments and improving communication with people with a disability.

Most areas of the UK have access to community learning disability teams; these teams are available for you to access and will be able to provide you with specialist information, resources and support. A key role of these teams is to advice and support primary care trusts in delivering annual health checks for people with an LD.

Activity 3.4 *Critical thinking*

Daniel is 30 years old and has Down's syndrome. He lives in supported accommodation with three other people with learning disabilities. Daniel relies on convenience foods the majority of the time, though his support worker is trying to improve his diet. He does not work and takes limited exercise; as a result he has been putting on weight. Daniel is attending his GP surgery for his annual health check. At this visit it is noted that his weight has increased and his BMI is 28 (it was 24 last year). This is concerning to Daniel's GP as his weight gain will increase his chances of developing Type 2 diabetes, heart disease, etc. Daniel's GP has asked the practice nurse to work with Daniel to reduce his weight.

How would you work with Daniel to improve his health by either changing his diet or increasing his exercise?

The RCN learning disability guidance, available from **www.rcn.org.uk** (and search for meeting the health needs of people with learning disabilities), is a resource that will help you with this question.

A brief outline answer is given at the end of the chapter.

By supporting Daniel to improve his health you will be able to increase his sense of autonomy and minimise his health complications in the future.

Conclusion

Having read through this chapter and worked through the activities you will have succeeded in increasing your knowledge and skills of health promotion in relation to the care and management of people living with an LTC. How you will use your knowledge and skills will depend on where you are working and your roles and responsibilities. Nevertheless, as a nurse you can increase the appropriateness of your health promotion by using the knowledge and skills developed in this chapter. By increasing your knowledge of health determinants and health promotion approaches you will be able to provide health promotion interventions that address the holistic nature of health. By understanding motivation in relation to health promotion and how to relate this to a person's readiness to change you will provide health promotion information appropriate for that person. In using a strategy like MI you will place the person at the centre of your interactions with them, ensuring that they are driving the health promotion.

Chapter summary

This chapter has provided you with an overview of the role of health promotion in the care and management of people living with an LTC. The importance of determinants of health and public health in relation to LTCs has been outlined. It has recognised the importance of health promotion in the care and management of people living with an LTC as this is a key message in recent health policy. It has focused on health promotion approaches and how to effect change in a person's health behaviour to enhance their health and wellbeing. Some specific behaviour change strategies that can be used in promoting health for people living with an LTC have been discussed and related to your clinical practice.

Activities: brief outline answers

Activity 3.2: Critical thinking (page 52)

- Genetic and biological factors – as Andrew has no known genetic illness this aspect does not have a negative effect on his current health. His COPD is influencing his current health, and due to the nature of this condition his symptoms are only likely to increase, resulting in poorer health, especially due to his recurrent chest infections. Through good management, Andrew's condition can improve his health by minimising symptoms.
- A person's characteristics and behaviours – Andrew manages to walk to his local shop to buy his food, though he does find this increasingly hard: this regular exercise is important for both management of his COPD and to encourage social interaction with others in his local community. The quality of Andrew's diet will depend on what food is available in his local shop, access to fresh fruit and veg, etc. Andrew also still smokes; this has the potential to have a huge negative effect on his health, especially in relation to his COPD, and could account for his recurrent chest infections. It should be noted that Andrew has tried to stop in the past, and was successful for a time, with the aim of trying to find out what prompted him to start again.
- A person's social and economic environment – Andrew enjoys the company that living in a sheltered housing complex gives him and this has the potential to have a positive effect on his overall health and wellbeing. Though his recent admissions to secondary care may have meant that he felt isolated from his friends, reintegrating Andrew back into the life of the sheltered housing complex will be important to maintain his level of socialisation. As a retired painter and decorator it is unlikely that Andrew will have access to a private pension and is probably relying on his state pension; the economic impact of this could impact on the choices he makes in relation to buying food, etc.
- A person's physical environment and social support network – Andrew is able to manage round his physical environment both inside and outside, in the local area, and this allows him to feel part of his local community and will have a positive effect on his health. Andrew felt very alone following the death of his wife, and he has now lost the support that the live-in warden gave him and may remind

him of the loss of his wife. How Andrew coped with the loss of his wife will influence how he copes with future losses. It is important for those involved in Andrew's care that they are aware of this as it may have a negative impact on his psychological wellbeing.

Activity 3.3: Critical thinking (page 57)

Examples are given here of how all health promotion approaches, except the social change approach, may be used to address Angela's sleepless nights.

- Medical – by recognising that fatigue can be a symptom of MS the medical approach may focus on assessing and managing Angela's fatigue; it may also focus on prescribing sedatives for Angela to take at night, though it may not necessarily address the underlying causes of this, for example, what is causing her sleepless nights?
- Educational – by answering any questions Angela may have and by providing specific information regarding her RRMS you will increase her understanding of her condition, and this may assist in alleviating some of her worries. By discussing local MS support groups with Angela you can provide her with another support mechanism and a source of information and advice.
- Behavioural – by focusing on changing Angela's behaviour when she wakes up you can assist her in improving the quality of her sleep. You might advise her to write down any specific questions that are troubling her – she can then address these during the day. Encouraging the use of relaxation to help Angela get back to sleep may also be appropriate, working with Angela to find out which type of relaxation method would suit her best. Providing Angela with a mechanism that she can use has the potential to empower her to take a more active role in managing her condition.
- Empowerment – by working with Angela to find out what her worries are when she wakes in the night, you can support her to find strategies that will both assist her in getting back to sleep (behaviour change approach) and will assist her in addressing some of the worries she may have (education approach). This approach has the potential to empower Angela and have a positive influence on her overall health and wellbeing. Increasing her knowledge and understanding of her condition and by providing her with strategies she can use to manage her condition, she will be able to take more control of her situation.

It is important that the impact of both these strategies is evaluated, and asking Angela to keep a sleep diary could be used as a means of evaluating the success or otherwise of your intervention.

Activity 3.4: Critical thinking (page 62)

Both you and the practice nurse will need to consider how you deliver information to Daniel in a format that he will understand. The British Institute of Learning Disabilities provides a range of books focusing on good health which includes titles on healthy eating and exercise. If providing written material, try to ensure that you address Daniel directly, e.g. playing football will help you lose weight and this is good for your heart. Using diagrams and pictures to illustrate the words will help reinforce the message. When discussing either healthy eating or exercise with Daniel speak clearly and allow Daniel time to answer. Provide your information in a positive way, e.g. don't say 'don't eat crisps every day', say 'have crisps on a Monday'. Always make sure that Daniel has understood the conversation, check at the end.

Working with Daniel's support worker and the local Community Learning Disability Team will ensure that Daniel is well supported.

Further reading

Bennett, C, Parry, J and Lawrence, Z (2009) Promoting Health in Primary Care. *Nursing Standard.* 23 (47), 48–56.
An overview of the role of health promotion in primary care.

Dixon, A (2008) *Motivation and Confidence: What Does it Take to Change Behaviour?* London: King's Fund.
A paper that discusses the role personal motivation and confidence have in relation to behaviour change.

Heathcote, J (2007) Using reminiscence: questions and answers. *Nursing and Residential Care.* 9 (7), 317–19
An article offering practical advice and answering frequently asked questions about reminiscence therapy.

Tribe, R, Lane, P and Heasum, S (2009) Working towards promoting positive mental health and wellbeing for older people from BME communities. *Working with Older People.* 13 (1), 35–40.
This article identifies some of the key issues to be addressed when promoting mental health in black and minority ethnic communities.

Useful websites

www.bild.org.uk/index.html
This is the home page of the British Institute of Learning Disabilities; it contains many interesting and useful resources in relation to health promotion.

www.continyou.org.uk/health_and_wellbeing/skilled_health
This is the home page of Skilled for Health, and contains many useful resources, information and case studies.

www.dh.gov.uk/en/PublicHealth/index.htm
This is the section of the Department of Health website that addresses public health; strategies that are currently in place to support public health can be accessed here.

www.dhsspsni.gov.uk/index/phealth.htm
This is the home page of the public health section of the Department of Health, Social Services and Public Safety. This area of the site has information on Public Health in Northern Ireland, including population projections, environmental health and public health policy.

www.healthscotland.com/
This is the home page for Scotland's health improvement agency; it contains information on all aspects of public health including population health information, health improvement programmes and available resources.

www.wales.nhs.uk/sitesplus/888/
The home page of Public Health Wales, this site contains information about all aspects of public health in Wales and the strategies and programmes in place.

Chapter 4
Self-management and empowerment in long term conditions

NMC Standards for Pre-registration Nursing Education

This chapter will address the following competencies:

Domain 1: Professional values

4. All nurses must work in partnership with service users, carers, families, groups, communities and organisations. They must manage risk, and promote health and wellbeing while aiming to empower choices that promote self-care and safety.

Domain 2: Communication and interpersonal skills

3.1 Adult nurses must promote the concept, knowledge and practice of self-care with people with acute and long term conditions, using a range of communication skills and strategies.

6. All nurses must take every opportunity to encourage health-promoting behaviour through education, role modelling and effective communication.

Domain 3: Nursing practice and decision-making

8. All nurses must provide educational support, facilitation skills and therapeutic nursing interventions to optimise health and wellbeing. They must promote self-care and management whenever possible, helping people to make choices about their healthcare needs, involving families and carers where appropriate, to maximise their ability to care for themselves.

8.1 Adult nurses must work in partnership with people who have long term conditions that require medical or surgical nursing, and their families and carers, to provide therapeutic nursing interventions, optimise health and wellbeing, facilitate choice and maximise self-care and self-management.

NMC Essential Skills Clusters

This chapter will address the following ESCs:

Cluster: Organisational aspects of care

9. People can trust the newly registered graduate nurse to treat them as partners and work with them to make a holistic and systematic assessment of their needs; to develop a personalised plan that is based on mutual understanding and respect for their individual situation, promoting health and wellbeing, minimising risk of harm and promoting their safety at all times.

continued opposite...

continued...

By the second progression point:

5. Contributes to care based on understanding how the different stages of an illness of disability can impact on patients and carers.

11. Where relevant, applies knowledge of age-related and condition-related anatomy, physiology and development when interacting with people.

By entry to the register:

14. Applies research-based evidence to practice.

16. Promotes health and wellbeing, self-care and independence by teaching and empowering people and carers to make choices in coping with the effects of treatment and the ongoing nature and likely consequences of a condition including death and dying.

10. People can trust the newly registered graduate nurse to deliver nursing interventions and evaluate their effectiveness against the agreed assessment and care plan.

By the second progression point:

1. Acts collaboratively with people and their carers, enabling and empowering them to take a shared and active role in the delivery and evaluation of nursing interventions.

By entry to the register:

6. Provides safe and effective care in partnership with people and their carers within the context of people's ages, conditions and developmental stages.

Chapter aims

After reading this chapter you will be able to:

- explain the role of empowerment in enabling self-management for people living with an LTC;

- identify the skills required to self-manage and how to develop these in people living with an LTC;

- understand the role that the Expert Patients Programme has in promoting self-management for people living with an LTC;

- recognise the role that self-management can play in the care of people living with dementia.

Introduction

There is no way you can avoid managing a chronic condition. If you do nothing but suffer, this is a management style. If you only take medication, this is another management style. If you choose to be a positive self-manager and undergo all the best treatments that healthcare professionals have to offer along with being proactive in your day to day management, this will lead you to live a healthy life.

(Lorig et al., 2006, page 1)

Living with the diagnosis of an LTC can have a profound impact on how individuals view themselves and their life. Until the time of diagnosis, they may have felt relatively in control of their life and future, but all this has changed with diagnosis. Now, they no longer feel they can control their life or future. The aim of self-management in the care and management of LTCs is to empower these individuals, and thereby enable them to maintain as much control over their life and future as they would like to have.

Self-management requires a change in a person's behaviour with regard to managing their LTC. Therefore it is likely that you will use some of the health promotion approaches and some of the behaviour change strategies discussed in Chapter 3 to support people with living with an LTC to self-manage. This is certainly what happened to James, who is living with epilepsy; this is how he describes his experience of living with epilepsy.

> When I was younger my parents were very supportive and tried to involve me in managing my condition, though mum was very protective, however I always felt different - people treating me differently, teacher and so on. When I went to university and I wasn't having any seizures I began to think maybe I can stop my medication. So I did, not only that but I started drinking quite a lot of alcohol, I was OK for a while then I had a seizure at night, thankfully one of my flatmates heard me and came in. That was that, straight off to A and E in an ambulance. I hadn't told anyone at university about my epilepsy, but I could see how frightened my flat mate had been. It was then I realised that I had to take control of my epilepsy, had to acknowledge it, yes it made me different but so what? Over the past few years I have worked hard with a counsellor who specialises in supporting young people with epilepsy. Things are improving, so much so that my counsellor has asked me if I would like to share my story with other young people with epilepsy.
>
> (James, mid-twenties, epilepsy)

In the quote above it is evident that James made a conscious decision to take control of his epilepsy rather than allowing his epilepsy to control him and his life. However, it should be recognised that not all people living with an LTC will feel able to, or want to, participate in their own self-management. For some people self-management of their LTC will not be an option. Bill is 79 and has chronic obstructive pulmonary disease; this is how he describes a visit to the hospital.

> They take your blood, there's no discussion, they're too busy, just a bloke with a machine. Then the nurse tells you there's no change this time, that things haven't altered. I don't want to know more. The GP - we work together - he tells me what to do - but he's the doctor, that's what he gets paid for, and what I paid in for, for all these years
>
> (Bill, 79, COPD (Corben and Rosen, 2005, page 3)

While it is evident that Bill does not want to be more involved in his care than he is, other people with LTCs may wish to self-manage their condition but are unable to. This could be for a variety of reasons, e.g. feeling that they are not being listened to, a lack of knowledge and understanding about their condition or their social situation. Engaging people like Bill in the self-management of their LTC requires you to address the underlying reasons for their reluctance to actively participate in their own self-management. By using the knowledge and skills discussed in Chapters 2 and 3 of this book, such as engaging in a therapeutic relationship and using effective communication skills, it will support you in being able to address these underlying reasons for their reluctance.

To support you in effectively accessing self-management strategies for people living with an LTC, including dementia, this chapter will develop your knowledge and skills in relation to self-management in the care and management of people living with an LTC. To do this, the chapter will discuss the importance of empowerment in self-management and how you can, through your actions, help to empower people living with an LTC. There will be a focus on what skills will help a person living with an LTC to become an effective self-manager, and how to develop those skills. The role of the Expert Patients Programme as a means of promoting self-management will be outlined. Finally, the importance of promoting self-management in dementia will be discussed, with some strategies for care being outlined. The terms self-care and self-management can be used to mean the same thing; for consistency the term self-management will be used throughout this chapter.

Policy review

As discussed in previous chapters, recent government policies across the UK have focused on improving the care and management of LTCs (DH, 2005; Department of Health and Social Services, 2007; Long Term Conditions Alliance Northern Ireland, 2008, NHS Scotland, 2009). In relation to the role of self-management each of these policy documents includes a specific mention of self-management:

- Department of Health (2005a): as part of quality requirement one: *providing good information and education benefits the person by improving opportunities for choice and levels of independence*;
- Department of Health and Social Services (2007): *increase self-management, independence and the participation of people with chronic conditions and their carers*;
- Long Term Conditions Alliance Northern Ireland (2008): *support for self-management training and other forms of structured, condition-specific patient education*;
- The Scottish Government Health Delivery Directorate Improvement Support Team (2009): High impact change 2: *we support people with long term conditions and their unpaid carers to be involved in person-centred care planning.*

In England the publication *Supporting People with Long Term Conditions: An NHS and Social Care Model to Support Local Innovation and Integration* (DH, 2005b) clearly stated the role that self-management would play in the care and management of LTC. Here the emphasis was placed on self-care being the cornerstone and largest section of the model. More recently, *Your Health, Your Way: A Guide to Long Term Conditions and Self-Care* (DH, 2009) clearly states the integral role self-management has in the day-to-day lives of people living with an LTC. Its aim is to raise awareness of the choices people living with an LTC have and supports people to exercise their choice to enable them to manage their life and not just their condition.

Empowerment as an ethos of care in LTCs

Empowerment is a process through which people gain greater control over decisions and actions affecting their health.

(World Health Organization, 1998)

Empowerment is not a specific strategy, approach, tool or skill that you can employ in the care and management of people living with an LTC. Rather, it is an **ethos** that will underpin your care and management of people living with an LTC. While you may not be directly involved in many of the self-management strategies available, for managing the care of people living with an LTC, e.g. Expert Patients Programme (EPP), you can play a significant role in encouraging and enabling people to either learn the skills of self-management or access programmes like the EPP. Empowerment therefore is discussed as an underlying element of your care and management and can be related to all aspects of this. For example, you should recognise that effective health promotion (see Chapter 3) has the potential to empower people living with an LTC to take more responsibility for managing their condition. To appreciate empowerment as part of the care and management of LTCs it is useful to have an awareness of its origins.

As a **philosophy,** empowerment began as a result of 'communities' or groups of people feeling oppressed and powerless. These 'communities' then empowered themselves by taking positive action and as a result became powerful and most importantly liberated. Examples of these include the civil rights movement in the USA, rights for disabled people and women's rights; these are examples of empowerment being used as social action. Paulo Freire (1921– 97) was a Brazilian theorist who worked with marginalised groups in Brazil promoting literacy. His seminal piece of work, *Pedagogy of the Oppressed* (1970), stated that it would be education that would enable oppressed groups to overcome their situation and regain their humanity (Smith, 1997, 2002). The fundamental principles of Freire's work still apply today and are relevant to empowering people living with an LTC. These principles are as follows.

- Dialogue – engaging in a therapeutic relationship with a person will allow for a framework of mutual respect and collaboration to develop.
- Understanding – using approaches like the transtheoretical model (DiClemente, 2007) and motivational interviewing will ensure that you understand a person's position and their values. Therefore the strategies you put in place will encompass those increasing their likelihood of success.
- Acknowledging those who do not have a voice – having an increased awareness of determinants of health, health inequalities and health literacy will support you in your role as a person's advocate.
- Experience – again through the use of an effective therapeutic relationship, and strategies like narrative-based care, you will be able to listen to and value the experience of the people who are living with an LTC (Smith, 1997, 2002).

The principles of Freire's work have also been used in the field of health literacy (Nutbeam, 2000; Kickbush, 2001), see also Chapter 3 of this book. Increasing a person's level of health literacy can be seen as a way of empowering them to be able to take control of their condition and play a more active role in managing their condition and their life. The focus of empowerment in this chapter relates to self-empowerment; however, it could be argued that in empowering an individual you are equipping them with the knowledge, skills and motivation to make not only personal changes but also broader community changes.

Activity 4.1   *Reflection*

Empowerment is about supporting a person to become more active and in control of their situation. Reflecting back on your life, personal and professional, think of a situation where you have been disempowered and answer the following questions.

- What was it about this situation that disempowered you?
- How did that make you feel?
- Were there any positive strategies, or was there anyone that helped you to be empowered in this situation?
- How might using how you felt being disempowered and some of the positive strategies that were used to assist you to empower people living with an LTC?

As the answers will be based on your own observations there is no outline answer at the end of this chapter.

The more traditional relationship in healthcare has focused on the healthcare professional as being in a position of power and the individual receiving the care being a passive recipient of this care. Empowering people living with an LTC to self-manage their condition challenges this relationship as people living with an LTC become partners in their care. It is therefore essential that you, as a healthcare professional, are aware of your beliefs and attitudes in relation to empowerment (Christensen and Hewlitt-Taylor, 2006); a question to ask yourself is:

- does your attitude towards the people you are caring for demonstrate to them that you value their contribution and decisions?

Your experience of being disempowered, subsequent reflection and response to the questions asked in Activity 4.1 will have informed how you respond to this question. Your response may also be influenced by other healthcare professionals you have worked with who you have seen value the contribution those living with an LTC can make to their care and management. By recognising and responding to your own experience of being disempowered, you will be better placed to promote empowerment for people living with an LTC. Toofany (2006) notes that as a nurse you cannot give a person 'empowerment'; they have to want to be empowered. However, there are certain attributes that you possess and actions that you take that can assist you in empowering people in your care (Table 4.1).

Your attributes	Your actions	Result in...
Kindness/cheerfulness	Taking the time to listen	Mutual trust
Experience	Taking the time to talk	Respect
Knowledge	Offering information	Open and genuine
Approachability	Answering questions	Communication

Table 4.1: Your attributes and actions that can result in empowerment

On the other hand there are some actions that are known to reduce empowerment; they are poor communication and showing a lack of respect for those in your care. There are other strategies, both on a one-to-one level and on a more strategic level, which can promote empowerment (Toofany, 2006) (Table 4.2).

Empowerment can be achieved by…	
On a one-to-one level	**On a strategic level**
Actively encouraging and supporting individuals to participate	Ensuring that individuals have a say in how healthcare services are delivered
Shifting the balance of power by reducing professional barriers	Promoting joint working and developing partnerships
Helping individuals to acquire decision-making skills	Moving towards a social model of healthcare and nursing
Enhancing communication strategies	Changing leadership culture
Valuing the knowledge of the community	Enhancing communication strategies
Increasing the sense of belonging, self-esteem and self-confidence	Valuing the knowledge of the community
Enhancing skills through education	Expanding programmes such as the EPP
	Setting up self-help groups

Table 4.2: Strategies to promote empowerment in the care and management of LTCs

Activity 4.2   *Reflection and critical thinking*

Using the same situation that you reflected on in Activity 4.1, the information in this chapter about empowerment and the resources in the further reading list, answer the following question.

• How should this situation have been managed to promote your empowerment?

As the answers will be based on your own observations there is no outline answer at the end of this chapter.

Corben and Rosen (2005) emphasise the importance of their being a good relationship between healthcare professionals and those living with an LTC. The aspects of this relationship echo those of the therapeutic relationship, as discussed in Chapter 2. These authors highlight the importance of listening, identifying the person's concern, allowing time for discussion and ensuring that there is a clear contribution by the person to the planning of their care. It is likely that your answer to Activity 4.2 included aspects of this. This is the same for people living with an LTC. It is through the use of an effective therapeutic relationship that people living with an LTC can be empowered to take a more active role in self-managing their condition.

Self-management in LTCs

Self-management is an important part of the care and management of people living with an LTC. It can be seen as an empowering right by many, although (as we have discussed) some people make a clear choice not to become more actively involved in managing their condition (Corben and Rosen, 2005). However, what is important is to know and understand what level of self-management a person living with an LTC is prepared and able to be involved in. For example, Bill's (see quote on page 68) level of engagement may relate to knowing the signs that indicate he is developing a chest infection and then knowing who to contact. Generally speaking, though, self-management is important both for the individual with an LTC and for the NHS. If someone with an LTC manages their condition themselves they may have relatively little contact with healthcare professionals. As mentioned in Chapter 1, 80% of GP consultations relate to people living with an LTC, but of those up to a quarter of consultations are for minor issues. Effective self-management has been shown to decrease demand on services including reducing GP consultations by up to 40% (DH, 2005c). Self-management that is clearly focused on the person living with an LTC, and on their needs, can enable them to participate in their care, empowering them to manage it and ensuring appropriate use of services. Crucial to the success of such an initiative is working with people to identify their own needs, and supporting them to make decisions about how they are going to meet them. There are some key skills that will enable them to do this effectively.

Effective skills for people living with an LTC to aid self-management

The skills that those living with an LTC should be developing, to support their self-management, relate to the following subsections (Lorig et al., 2006; Carrier, 2009).

Skills needed to manage their LTC

Any LTC requires the person living with it to learn to do new things. This includes knowledge of the condition and how to manage the symptoms: for example medication management, changes to their diet or coping with side-effects of chemotherapy. Living with an LTC may require more interactions with healthcare services, so it is important that the person knows how to access services.

Skills needed to maintain their normal life

The diagnosis of an LTC does not mean that the person's life has to stop. Managing symptoms, responding to changes and recognising a deterioration in their condition are important factors in maintaining a normal life. It is also important for individuals to have an awareness of how their lifestyle choices can affect their condition.

Skills needed to manage the emotional aspect of living with their LTC

Being diagnosed and living with an LTC can result in a person experiencing emotional changes, some of which can be negative. Learning new skills to develop their emotional intelligence (see Chapter 2) will support them to manage this aspect of their care.

Working with a person living with an LTC to develop these skills will promote self-management, enabling that person to navigate their way through the challenges of living with their LTC (Lorig et al., 2006; Carrier, 2009).

Activity 4.3   *Critical thinking*

Using one of the following case scenarios (see website: **www.learningmatters.co.uk/nursing** for full case scenarios):

* Andrew, aged 75, a widower and living with COPD;
* Angela, aged 28, married, has one son and living with RRMS;
* Frazer, aged 42, married, has one daughter and living with Type 1 diabetes;

outline what skills would be beneficial for them to learn to enable them to manage the following aspects of living with their specific LTC:

* dealing with their LTC;
* maintaining their normal life;
* managing the emotional aspect of living with their LTC.

A brief outline answer is given at the end of the chapter.

Your Health, Your Way (DH, 2009) is designed to help people with LTCs to develop a greater sense of control over their condition. Self-management is categorised into five areas: information, skills and knowledge training, tools and self-monitoring devices, healthy lifestyle choices and support networks. The skills identified above support these categories. So, for example, in Activity 4.3 Fraser's foot care falls into the category of knowledge and training while Angela's planned return to work falls into support networks. Some of the skills outlined in Activity 4.3 also require the person with the LTC to be able to problem-solve and plan a course of action, for example how can Andrew recognise when he is developing a chest infection. Individuals might find this quite daunting, so here are some strategies to support you help people with self-management.

Developing a person's ability to self-manage their LTC

Action planning and problem solving have been identified as examples of strategies that can be used to promote effective self-care in people living with an LTC (Lorig et al., 2006: Carrier, 2009). Action planning has been used successfully in the management of asthma and COPD. The following research summary focuses on action planning as a strategy for people living with asthma and COPD to be able to recognise and self-treat an exacerbation.

Research summary

Action planning is recommended as a strategy to use in the management of asthma (Gibson and Powell, 2004; SIGN, 2009). The focus of action planning in asthma has been on providing a set of instructions for a person living with asthma to use in the management of an acute exacerbation. Gibson and Powell (2004) undertook a review of the evidence base in relation to effectiveness of individualised action plans in the early detection and treatment of an asthma exacerbation. An individualised plan is written,

continued opposite...

continued...

taking into account the person's underlying asthma severity and their current treatment regime. They identified 26 randomised controlled trials that had evaluated action plans as part of asthma self-management. Of these, 17 action plans were classified as being complete as they contained individualised information that included the following:

- when to increase treatment (including medications);
- how to increase treatment (including medications);
- for how long;
- when to seek medical assistance.

They found nine action plans that were either incomplete (they did not specify the use of inhaled corticosteroids (ICS) as an early intervention) or non-specific (they included general information). Their results indicated that individualised action plans with two to four action points and using both ICS and oral corticosteroids (OCS) improved health outcomes. Action points are activated when a certain level of symptom or lung function is reached, e.g. the first action point may be when a person's peak expiratory flow rate is at 70–85% of their best. As an exacerbation of asthma consists of both airflow obstruction and airway inflammation, appropriate treatment may recommend increasing both ICS and OCS. They also noted that action points based on a person's best peak expiratory flow (PEF) rate improved health outcomes, whereas action points based on percentage predicted PEF did not. Where a person's best PEF was used there were reductions in hospital admissions, attendance at accident and emergency and improved PEF. Their review concluded that the use of individualised action plans based on a person's best PEF, using between two and four action points and recommending both the use of ICS and OCS consistently improved health outcomes.

For examples of action plans access the following websites: **www.sign.ac.uk/pdf/ sign101.pdf** (British Thoracic Society and Scottish Intercollegiate Guidelines Network, 2009) and **www.patient.co.uk/doctor/Asthma-Action-Plans.htm**.

Some preliminary work has been undertaken in relation to using action plans to manage exacerbations of COPD. In 2005, Turnock and colleagues undertook a systematic review of the Cochrane Database to assess the effectiveness of action plans in the management of COPD. Their results concluded that there was evidence of action plans having a positive effect on self-management. This primarily related to their ability to recognise a deterioration in their condition and to their ability to self-start treatment, e.g. commencing antibiotics or steroids. The Canadian Thoracic Society has an action plan for COPD that can be accessed via their website: **www.copdguidelines.ca/resources-ressources_e. php#actionplan**.

The focus of this section is about action planning and problem solving being used to support people living with an LTC to self-manage their condition on a day-to-day basis. Discussing action planning and problem solving with people living with an LTC, identifying how these can help them to self-manage and working with them in the initial stages have the potential to increase their sense of confidence and self-efficacy in relation to self-management of their LTC. The process of action planning and problem solving begins with the person identifying what they want to accomplish: their goal (Frazer would like to minimise the risk of developing further foot ulcers). The purpose of action planning is to break down that person's goal into smaller tasks (e.g. how is Frazer going to achieve this; what does he have to do?). Therefore, while the overall goal might be quite large, the action plan breaks it down into manageable pieces, enabling the person to see that they are working towards their overall goal. For an action plan to be successful it should relate to something the person wants to do. Also, Lorig et al. (2006) state it should:

- be reasonable – is this something that the person can expect to achieve in a reasonable time, such as in a week or two;
- be behaviour-specific – giving the person an identified behaviour to address, something they can actually see changing (e.g. rather than saying 'losing weight' say 'no eating after dinner');
- answer the following questions: What is the person is going to do? How often are they going to do this? When they are going to do this?
- inspire confidence – how confident is the person that they are going to achieve this? They could rate this on a scale of one to ten, one being no confidence and ten being most confident. If a person rates their confidence below seven, they should asks themselves why their confidence is low and review their action plan in a way that will increase their likelihood of success.

When completing an action plan a person may experience problems that affect their ability to achieve what they had set out to do. This could be for a variety of reasons: the overall goal was unrealistic, the action plan was too ambitious or their condition deteriorates. What is important here is that the person does not give up but finds ways to solve the problem that is preventing them in reaching their goal. This could take the form of reviewing their goal or giving themselves longer to complete their action plan. Supporting people living with an LTC to find solutions to their problems will increase their knowledge and understanding of their LTC, increase the skills required to manage their LTC and increase their self-efficacy in managing their LTC.

Case study: Frazer

Frazer is 42 and is living with Type 1 diabetes. In the past he has not always managed his diabetes well. This has resulted in Frazer developing diabetic polyneuropathy: he has an ulcer on his foot that is slow to heal. He sees the practice nurse regularly to have this dressed, and during one of his consultations he asks what he can do to prevent further problems with his feet. He would like to minimise the risk of further ulcers developing. The practice nurse works with Frazer to devise an action plan to help him achieve this.

As long as Frazer has ongoing foot problems it would be advisable for him to continue to use an action plan addressing foot hygiene. To support this action plan it may also be necessary to discuss diabetic polyneuropathy with Frazer. Diabetic polyneuropathy is caused when there is damage to the peripheral nervous system. High levels of blood glucose cause biochemical changes that cause destruction of the nerves associated with damage to blood vessels also due to high blood glucose levels. Given that both motor and sensory nerves are affected this can affect Frazer's movement and his ability to feel sensations such as heat, etc. This will result in Frazer experiencing one or more of the following symptoms:

- *numbness and tingling in his feet and hands;*
- *burning, shooting or stabbing pains;*
- *loss of coordination in the affected area;*
- *muscle weakness.*

Action Plan

Goal: to minimise the risk of further foot ulceration through appropriate foot care

Aim: to monitor my feet for signs of change – every morning this week I will:

- *examine my feet assessing colour, swelling, breaks in the skin and pain or numbness;*
- *wash and dry my feet carefully;*
- *apply moisturiser to my feet.*

This week I will avoid:

- *walking around barefoot;*
- *hot water bottles, hot baths, etc.*

This week I will remember to:

- *ensure my socks and shoes are well fitting.*

This week I will be aware of the danger of:

- *skin removal, e.g. corns.*

What to do if anything changes:

- *if I notice any changes in my feet, especially my ulcer, I am to notify healthcare professionals immediately to ensure appropriate treatment and management.*

How confident am I that I will achieve this? 8 out of 10

Day of the week	Achieved	Any comments
Monday	*Yes*	*Inspected my feet today, used a mirror to help me check the soles of my feet, remembered to dry and apply moisturiser after my shower*
Tuesday	*Yes*	*As Monday*
Wednesday	*Yes*	*As Monday, did notice that some of my socks were a bit worn, off to get some new ones tomorrow*
Thursday	*Yes*	*Slept in this morning, no shower today but did inspect them, wash, dry and moisturise them tonight*
Friday	*Yes*	*As Monday*
Saturday	*No*	*Went swimming today with Fiona, too busy making sure she was dried and dressed, forgot to dry my feet properly and put on moisturiser*
Sunday	*Yes*	*Noticed that the area round my dressing was slightly red and appeared swollen. Contacted NHS Direct, advised to attend out of hours service, antibiotics prescribed, appointment with practice nurse to be arranged.*

Activity 4.4   *Critical thinking*

Case study: Andrew

Andrew is 75 and is living with COPD. He has had several recent chest infections that have meant he has been admitted into secondary care. At a recent consultation Andrew expressed concern about his condition and was asked what he could do to help manage his COPD better. His consultant discussed the importance of maintaining his fitness levels as this would help control his breathlessness and maintain his current lung function. Andrew is keen to do this but is unsure how to begin; the respiratory nurse specialist is visiting him to assist him to make a plan to achieve this. You are spending the day with her and visit Andrew with her. Prior to the visit you read up on exercise and COPD, especially pursed lip breathing and arm and leg exercises.

How would you compile an action plan, with Andrew, incorporating pursed lip breathing and leg and arm exercises to maintain and if possible increase his lung function?

To find out more about pursed lip breathing, take a look at the video clip on **www. youtube.com/watch?=jFqrWVeskR0**.

Now that you have compiled an action plan for Andrew have a go at compiling one for Angela to address one of the needs outlined in Activity 4.3.

A brief outline answer is given at the end of the chapter for Andrew; however, there is no outline answer for Angela as your answer will depend on what aspect of Angela's self-management you address.

As you can see from Activity 4.4, successful self-management relies on the person who is living with the LTC being able to identify specific goals they would like to achieve and planning and implementing a course of action to enable them to succeed. However, it should be recognised that for some people there may be times where some goals are unachievable, for example if Frazer were to develop a wound infection. In this situation it is important to support Frazer in compiling an action plan to address his infection so that he will be able to return to his first goal. Alternatively it may be appropriate to find other goals that are more achievable for the individual at that time. This flexible positive approach will focus on what the person can do rather than what they cannot do.

The aim of action planning, as discussed above, is to enable the person living with an LTC to successfully self-manage their condition. However, you will have seen that some of the time people living with an LTC will require intervention from other healthcare professionals, e.g. physiotherapist for pulmonary rehabilitation, or podiatrist for foot care. Self-management, therefore, is not about the person living with the LTC managing their care in isolation. It is about the person living with the LTC working with members of the healthcare team, accessing relevant information and education and then using what they have learned to manage their condition in the way that best suits their lifestyle (Lorig et al., 2006).

A strategy to suppport self-management

So far the focus of this chapter has been on how you, in your role as a nurse, can empower and support people living with an LTC to manage their own condition. However, there are other members of the healthcare team and other organisations who can help promote self-management for people living with an LTC.

The Expert Patients Programme

The aim of the EPP is, through self-management, to provide people, living with an LTC, with the knowledge, tools and skills to effectively manage their LTC and maintain control of their condition and life. The concept behind the EPP is that people living with an LTC very often know and understand their condition, on a day-to-day basis, better than the healthcare professionals. Therefore the idea was that a partnership would develop between the person with the LTC and the healthcare professionals. The professionals would be responsible for the diagnosis, monitoring and management of the condition, through tests and treatment. The person living with the LTC would be responsible for adapting their lifestyle, taking prescribed medication and reporting changes to maximise their health and wellbeing (Phillips, 2009). The course tutors are all lay people, living with an LTC, who have completed an EPP themselves and have undergone a four-day tutor training course.

Courses are free and run over six weeks. The tutors do not provide all the answers; instead, the process of the course is to support those participating to identify their own requirements and to look at ways to address those. This is done through the use of goal setting, action planning and problem solving. The course addresses the following areas (Phillips, 2009):

- dealing with pain and extreme tiredness (fatigue);
- coping with feelings of depression, fear and frustration;
- relaxation techniques and exercise;
- healthy eating;
- communicating with family, friends and professionals;
- planning for the future.

An evaluation of the EPP, through the use of a randomised controlled trial (Rogers et al., 2006), demonstrated it to be cost-effective. It was also found to improve participants' wellbeing, self-efficacy and communication with healthcare professionals. The EPP Community Interest Group (CIG) now runs many other courses, including:

- new beginnings – a course for people affected by a mental health condition;
- looking after me and caring with confidence – courses for carers (see Chapter 2 for more information);
- substance and alcohol misuse – a course for people recovering from substance or alcohol misuse;
- supporting parents programme – a course for parents of a child living with an LTC;
- staying positive – a workshop for people aged between 12 and 18 who are living with an LTC;
- learning difficulties course – a course for people living with a learning disability to manage their health better;

- courses addressing specific aspects of living with an LTC – COPD and breathlessness, persistent pain programme and X-PERT diabetes course.

People living with an LTC can either apply to attend an Expert Patients Programme themselves or they can be referred by a member of the healthcare team.

Self-management for people living with dementia

The British Psychological Society (BPS) and Gaskell in 2007 published *Dementia: The NICE–SCIE Guideline on Supporting People with Dementia and their Carers in Health and Social Care.* This document clearly recognises the role of self-management for those living with dementia and their carers. Section 7 of these guidelines focuses on the therapeutic interventions that will maintain function of these. Providing strategies that promote independence is recognised as being important. People with dementia often find that their level of ability to carry out their activities of daily living (ADL) deteriorates more than the disease alone would account for. If you are involved in the care and management of people living with dementia, it is therefore important that you provide opportunities for individuals to maintain an active life. There is limited research available on this; however, a study in 2005 by Barclay et al. evaluated the Partnering with your Doctor programme in California. The aim of this programme was to provide education and information to enable both people living with dementia and their carers to improve their level of self-management. The researchers found that participants on the programme had increased levels of confidence, participated more in consultations and were able to work effectively with members of the healthcare team to improve their overall health. The guidelines published by the BPS in 2007 recognise the following areas of good practice in promoting self-management in dementia care.

Communication

People living with dementia should have their hearing and vision checked regularly and professionals should ensure that, when communicating, they take into consideration the individual's ability to communicate. Verbal communication should match the person's level of cognitive ability. Adapting your rate of speech, tone and words used to find the ones that get the best response from the person is also important. Memory books containing images and simple statements can be used to aid communication and memory recall. A memory book may include a family photograph with the names of the people in the photograph next to them. They can also be used when the same question is asked repeatedly, by providing a simple answer to the question through words and pictures. Carers may be advised to keep a diary of the following: changes in memory ability, drastic mood changes, unusual behaviour, health related changes to sleep, appetite, etc., and any health complaints of the person (Barclay et al., 2005). All this information can then be used to support the person living with dementia and to improve communication with healthcare professionals.

Activities of daily living (ADL) skill training and activity planning

Both ADL skill training and activity planning are areas of promoting self-management for people living with dementia that are coordinated by occupational therapists and physiotherapists.

However, as a nurse working in a multidisciplinary team, having an awareness and understanding of these areas of dementia care will improve the level of care and support you can provide. Both ADL skill training and activity planning identifies the strengths of the person living with dementia and the challenges they face. ADL skill training involves assessing the person's ability, level of impairment and ability to perform everyday tasks. A training programme is then implemented, taking into consideration the person's physical, psychological and cognitive ability. By increasing the range of activities the person is able to undertake, the aim of the programme is to maximise the health and wellbeing of both the person with dementia and their carer. ADL skill training has been shown to promote independence in a person's ability to undertake personal care tasks; it has also been shown to reduce carer stress. The programme includes graded assistance; this means that the carer gives the least amount of assistance needed in order for a person to complete the task. Assistance may take the form of verbal cues, visual cues, demonstration and some physical assistance (BPS, 2007). In activity planning by focusing on the interests, preferences and life histories of people living with dementia the Pool Activity Level (PAL) instrument can be used to plan meaningful activities. Using PAL will ensure that the activities are presented to the person with dementia at the appropriate level (**www.jpa-dementia.co.uk/index.php**).

Assistive technology

Assistive technology refers to equipment that may increase the range of activities, the independence and wellbeing of people living with a disability, either physical or cognitive. These include devices such as home blood pressure monitoring devices, blood glucose monitoring equipment and watches for cardiovascular monitoring. Assistive technology can be used to support people living with an LTC to self-manage. It also includes adaptive aids, environmental modifications and telecare. It is important to keep the technology simple and appropriate to a person's level of need. For example, if a person is falling, find out why. Falls could be due to poor footwear, loose rugs or poor lighting. In this situation low level technology such as lighting that is activated by movement can help reduce the risk of a person falling by ensuring their environment is well lit. Using well-positioned visual prompts (either words or pictures) around the house will assist a person with dementia to move around their home safely. Examples might include a picture of a bed on the bedroom door, or a notice saying 'tea and coffee' on a kitchen cupboard. Using memory aids such as calendars, diaries and a schedule of their daily routine can all improve a person's self-management and independence.

Telecare is the delivery of care to people living in their own home via computers and telecommunications systems. It involves a range of services including household safety, such as carbon monoxide detectors, fire or smoke detectors and flood detectors. While these services can be useful, they rely on the person understanding what the alarm is and what it means. Therefore assessment of the person's ability to recognise and interpret the alarm is important. Telecare also includes services to ensure personal safety such as fall detectors and bed or chair occupancy sensors. Fall detectors can sense a serious fall and will raise the alarm at the monitoring centre; the monitoring centre will then contact the registered emergency contact number, ensuring that the incident is responded to. Bed or chair occupancy sensors can be used at night; they can be programmed to switch on lights, minimising the risk of falls, an important aspect to consider if the person is known to experience nocturnal wandering. Many of the devices do not require the person with dementia to remember where they are or how to use them. It should be remembered though that devices such as the fall detector rely on the person putting in on every day; this may not be suitable for people living on their own. It is clear that assistive technology has a role to play in promoting the independence of people living with dementia; however, it should be used alongside other forms of care such as a day hospital and support groups, and not as a substitute for these.

Activity 4.5   *Reflection*

Using a model of reflection, such as the one by Gibbs (1988) and the following questions as prompts, reflect back on a situation when you have cared for a person with dementia.

- Were any of the areas of good practice identified in this chapter used in the care and management of the person with dementia?
- If not, then why was this?
- If yes, then why was this?
- What areas of good practice could have been used to promote independence for the person?
- How will this influence your practice in the future?

Using a model of reflection will assist you to structure your reflection, ensuring that you stay focused on a specific topic. Using the questions listed will further increase your level of analysis of the situation, developing your ability to critically analyse your practice and the practice of colleagues.

As the answers will be based on your own observations and discussions there is no outline answer at the end of this chapter.

Conclusion

Having read through this chapter and undertaken the activities you will have developed your knowledge and skills about the role of self-management in LTCs and how to empower individuals to take a more active role in managing their LTC. How you use the information in this chapter will depend on where you are working and your current responsibilities. However, in your role as a nurse, you can improve a person's self-management by developing the skills required to become an effective self-manager. You can utilise goal setting, action planning and problem solving to enable a person with an LTC to regain control of their condition and their life. By having an increased awareness of some of the strategies available to support self-management you will provide holistic care for those living with an LTC.

Self-management in dementia is an important aspect of their care and management; using the information provided in this chapter, you will enhance your care of this group of people.

Self-management is not about the person living with the LTC managing their care in isolation. It is about the person living with the LTC working with members of the healthcare team, accessing relevant information and education and then using that information to manage their condition in the way that best suits their life (Lorig et al., 2006).

Chapter summary

This chapter has provided you with an overview of the role of self-management in the care and management of people living with an LTC, a key element of recent health policy. It has outlined the importance of empowerment to promote a person's self-efficacy, a crucial aspect of successful self-management. There has been a clear focus on the person with the LTC and supporting them to develop their skills in relation to self-management. Specific ways in which to do this have been discussed and applied to your clinical practice. The importance of self-management in dementia has also been discussed with some specific areas of good practice being identified.

Activities: brief outline answers

Activity 4.3 (page 74)

Andrew

- Skills to manage his LTC – to include: medication management and effective use of his inhalers; how to recognise when he is developing a chest infection; increasing his confidence during consultations; pulmonary rehabilitation and healthy eating.
- Skills to maintain his normal life – to include: pacing himself when carrying out self-care to minimise his breathlessness and using the same technique when he goes shopping; recognise the impact his smoking is having.
- Skills to manage the emotional aspect of living with his LTC – to include: Andrew recognising the long-lasting impact of Elizabeth's death and planning for his future care needs, e.g. palliative care.

Angela

- Skills to manage her LTC – to include: management of fatigue and how to minimise this; increase her knowledge of other symptoms and how to recognise an exacerbation of her RRMS.
- Skills to maintain her normal life – to include: possible adaptations to house should she experience difficulties in mobilising; maintaining her role as mother and wife and planning for her return to work.
- Skills to manage the emotional aspect of living with her LTC – to include: relaxation techniques to manage her anxiety.

Frazer

- Skills to manage his LTC – to include: foot care and hygiene due to his ulcer; regular eye checks; blood glucose monitoring and effective insulin administration technique and healthy eating.
- Skills to maintain his normal life – to include: appropriate choice of footwear: raising his awareness of the impact of smoking and maintaining his part time status at work.
- Skills to manage the emotional aspect of living with his LTC – to include: managing his emotional response to non-healing foot ulcer and to his smoking.

Activity 4.4 (page 78)

Andrew

It is important that Andrew is aware of the benefits of maintaining his fitness levels. For people living with COPD anxiety can cause them to limit their exercise, and this in turn reduces their lung function and increases their breathlessness. Exercise has been shown to reduce symptoms in people with COPD. Andrew may require a different action plan each week or two weeks depending on how well he is increasing his exercise. A first action plan for Andrew, covering week one, might include the following.

Action plan

Goal: to maintain my level of lung function and to increase it if possible

Aim: to take more exercise and maintain my lung function:
Walking to my local shop every day in the morning:

- *I will remember to expect some breathlessness when I am walking and that this is normal.*
- *Be aware that cold weather might make my breathing more difficult.*

Every day before I go for a walk I will:

- *Do my pursed lip breathing for 10 mins – I will breathe in through my nose, move my abdominal muscles out, I will then breathe out through my mouth with my lips pursed and make a hissing sound. I will make sure that I breathe out for twice as long as I breathe in*

Carrying out exercises at home twice a week after lunch to include:

- *Knee extension – I will sit with my feet slightly apart and breathe out as I straighten my knee and raise my lower leg. I will then breathe in as I lower my leg. I will do this five times with each leg.*
- *Arm extension – sitting down with my arms by my side I will breathe out as I raise my arm to shoulder height. I will keep my arm straight, I will breathe out as I lower my arm.*

What to do if anything changes: *If my breathlessness gets worse, I am to take a note of any other symptoms and to contact the respiratory nurse specialist for advice.*

How confident am I that I will achieve this? 7 out of 10.

Day of the week	Achieved	Any comments
Monday		
Tuesday		
Wednesday		
Thursday		
Friday		
Saturday		
Sunday		

Further reading

Corben, S and Rosen, R (2005) *Self-management for Long-term Conditions: Patient's Perspectives on the Way Ahead.* London: King's Fund.
This reviews individuals' perceptions about self-management and sets out three key areas for development.

Department of Health (2005c) *Self Care – A Real Choice: Self Care Support – A Practical Option.* London: Department of Health.
Useful and practical information about promoting self-management for people with LTCs.

Social Care Institute for Excellence and National Institute for Health and Clinical Excellence (2007) *Dementia: the NICE–SCIE Guideline on Supporting People with Dementia and their Carers in Health and Social Care.* London: British Psychological Society.

Provides comprehensive guidance for the care and management of people living with dementia.

Useful websites

www.expertpatients.co.uk/
The home page of the EPP contains information about all the courses they run.

www.informationprescription.info/index.html
The home page of information prescriptions, external links to the information prescription services where you can create your own information prescription. This service is also available via the NHS Choices website.

www.ltcani.org.uk/index.asp
The home page of the Long Term Conditions Alliance Northern Ireland, a good source of relevant information relating to Northern Ireland.

www.ltcas.org.uk/index.html
The home page of the Long Term Conditions Alliance Scotland, a good source of information, including 'Gaunyersel!' their self-management strategy for LTCs.

www.nationalvoices.org.uk/
National voices is a group of organisations that campaign for change in health and social care. This home page has links to policy and campaign and service user involvement.

www.nhs.uk/Planners/Yourhealth/Pages/Yourhealth.aspx
The home page for Your Health, Your Way, providing lots of relevant information in relation to courses and support, healthy living, etc., in relation to LTCs.

www.scie.org.uk/publications/dementia/about.asp
This website focuses on information to support people living with dementia to maintain their independence.

Chapter 5
Quality of life and symptom management in long term conditions

NMC Standards for Pre-registration Nursing Education

This chapter will address the following competencies:

Domain 3: Nursing practice and decision-making

1. All nurses must use up-to-date knowledge and evidence to assess, plan, deliver and evaluate care, communicate findings, influence change and promote health and best practice. They must make person-centred, evidence-based judgements and decisions, in partnership with others involved in the care process, to ensure high quality care. They must be able to recognise when the complexity of clinical decisions requires specialist knowledge and expertise, and consult or refer accordingly.

1.1 Adult nurses must be able to recognise and respond to the needs of all people who come into their care including babies, children and young people, pregnant and post-natal women, people with mental health problems, people with physical disabilities, people with learning disabilities, older people, and people with long term problems such as cognitive impairment.

NMC Essential Skills Clusters

This chapter will address the following ESCs:

Cluster: Nutrition and food management

27. People can trust the newly registered graduate nurse to assist them to choose a diet that provides an adequate nutritional and fluid intake.

By the second progression point:

1. Under supervision helps people to choose healthy food and fluid in keeping with their personal preferences and cultural needs.

By entry to the register:

9. Discusses in a non-judgemental way how diet can improve health and the risks associated with not eating appropriately.

Cluster: Medicines management

34. People can trust the newly registered graduate nurse to work within legal and ethical frameworks that underpin safe and effective medicines management.

continued opposite...

continued...

By the second progression point:

2. Demonstrates an understanding of the types of prescribing, types of prescribers and methods of supply.

35. People can trust the newly registered graduate nurse to work as part of a team to offer holistic care and a range of treatment options of which medicines may form a part.

By the second progression point:

1. Demonstrates awareness of a range of commonly recognised approaches to managing symptoms, for example, relaxation, distraction and lifestyle advice.

Chapter aims

After reading this chapter you will be able to:

*   explain what quality of life (**QoL**) is and how it can be measured and its importance in the care and management of LTCs;
*   appreciate the importance of maintaining quality of life of people living with an LTC and where appropriate those caring for them;
*   recognise the role the nursing process has in effective symptom management;
*   explain the relevance of medicines management in the successful management of symptoms in people living with an LTC.

Introduction

Chronic illnesses come with symptoms. These symptoms are signals from the body that something unusual is happening. They cannot be seen by others, are often difficult to describe to others, and are usually unpredictable.

(Lorig et al., 2006, page 39)

Many symptoms of LTCs can be managed and minimised by person-centred health promotion and health education and by effective self-management. However, for some people living with an LTC their disease progression is marked out by changing, and often worsening, signs and symptoms. A sign is something that is noticed by other people and is generally objective and can be seen, heard, felt or measured. For example, a daughter may notice her mother becoming increasingly forgetful, and an assessment of this using the Mini Mental State Examination confirms reduced cognitive impairment. A symptom is noticed by the person with the LTC, is generally subjective and cannot always be measured, seen, heard or felt. For example, a person living with eczema may experience a severe itch, though on observation there may be no noticeable cause of the itch. A feature of an LTC may be both a sign and a symptom, e.g., increased pain in a venous leg ulcer is a symptom for the person with the leg ulcer but is a sign to the nurse that infection is present. The ability of a person living with an LTC to recognise relevant signs and symptoms and to effectively manage these improves their health outcome and quality of life and is one of the key aspects in the promotion of self-management in LTCs.

Activity 5.1   *Evidence-based practice and research*

Research the following LTCs: coronary heart disease (CHD), rheumatoid arthritis (RA) and Parkinson's disease (PD) and answer the following questions.

- What are the main signs and symptoms of these LTCs?
- Why do these signs and symptoms occur?
- Briefly describe how these signs and symptoms can be managed.

Some useful resources:

- your preferred applied anatomy and physiology text books;
- **www.cks.nhs.uk/home** – this is a useful website for healthcare professionals working in primary care, and provides evidence-based information on managing common conditions seen in primary care;
- **www.patient.co.uk/** – this comprehensive website contains information on many health conditions.

A brief outline answer is given at the end of the chapter.

As you can see from Activity 5.1 there are many signs and symptoms that require effective management when caring for people living with an LTC. Many people will experience more than one symptom and will be taking medication and using other therapeutic interventions to manage these. Previous chapters in this book have recognised the importance of engaging in a therapeutic relationship, the role of effective health promotion and the importance of self-management in the care and management of LTCs. All of these can be used to support effective symptom management in the care and management of LTCs. If someone with CHD smokes, health promotion will play a part in supporting them to change their health behaviour. Working with someone living with RA and helping them to formulate an action plan to ensure they are taking regular exercise will enable them to self-manage their condition. If you are caring for a person with PD, engaging in and ensuring an effective therapeutic relationship is maintained will enable you to pick up subtle changes that may indicate they are becoming depressed. Building on the knowledge and skills you have developed while working through the previous chapters, this chapter will help you to improve the quality of life quality of life of people living with an LTC through effective medicines management, nutritional support and symptom management. This chapter supports the development of your knowledge, skills and attributes in relation to quality of life and effective symptom management. The nursing process will be used to structure the symptom management discussed.

Policy review

The policies previously discussed in this book do not explicitly mention symptom management in relation to the care and management of LTCs (DH, 2005; Department of Health, Social

Services and Public Safety (DHSSPS), 2007; Long Term Conditions Alliance Northern Ireland (LTCANI), 2008; The Scottish Government Health Delivery Directorate Improvement Support Team, 2009). It should be noted, however, that one of the overarching themes within these policies is the improvement in quality of life for people living with an LTC. Along with health promotion and self-management, effective symptom management can help to achieve this. Specific information on the treatment and management of individual LTCs is available via the relevant NSF or National Institute for Health and Clinical Excellence (NICE), Scottish Intercollegiate Guidelines Network (SIGN) and DHSSPS publications. Examples of these include:

* CHD – *National Service Framework for Coronary Heart Disease* (DH, 2000b), *Heart Disease Guidelines* (SIGN, 2007), *Service Framework for Cardiovascular Health and Wellbeing* (DHSSPS, 2009a);
* RA – *Management of Early Rheumatoid Arthritis* (SIGN, 2000), *Rheumatoid Arthritis: The management of rheumatoid arthritis in adults* (NICE, 2009c);
* respiratory disease – *Chronic Obstructive Pulmonary Disease: Management of Chronic Obstructive Pulmonary Disease in Adults in Primary and Secondary Care (partial update)* (NICE, 2010), *British Guidelines on the Management of Asthma: A National Clinical Guideline* (SIGN, 2009), *Service Framework for Respiratory Health and Wellbeing* (DHSSPS, 2009b).

Quality of life in LTCs

Quality of life is the value assigned to the duration of life as modified by the social opportunities, perceptions, functional states and impairments that are influenced by disease, injuries, treatment or policies.

(Patrick and Erickson, 1993)

Quality of life is the degree to which a person enjoys the important possibilities of his or her life.

(Raphael et al., 1999)

The above quotes define quality of life in very different ways. The first one focuses on the impact health (health-related QoL), and loss of health, has on the quality of a person's life. The second one addresses QoL in relation to a person's opportunities and limitations and their enjoyment of their life, by its nature it is a more holistic definition. As you can see, defining QoL can be problematic depending on what you are assessing it against. There are many factors that influence your QoL, many of which can be related back to the determinants of health discussed in Chapter 3. The factors that influence and affect your QoL may be different from that of your friends, family, colleagues and those in your care. Over your lifetime it is likely that some of the factors influencing and affecting your QoL will change. It is this subjective aspect of QoL that makes it challenging to measure and quantify. However, it is also likely that there are some key factors that are important to your QoL whatever age and stage of your life.

Measuring quality of life in LTCs

To assist you in your care of people living with an LTC it is helpful to understand how QoL can be measured. There are many QoL assessment scales available: some focus on specific LTCs; e.g. the QoL after myocardial infarction (QLMI) (Valenti et al., 1996) and the Warwick–Edinburgh

Mental Well-being Scale (WEMWBS) (Tennant et al., 2007). Some are generic and can be used across a range of LTCs. Generic scales are useful as they allow you, as a nurse, to undertake an initial assessment of a person's QoL, which may or may not result in referrals being made to other members of the healthcare team. One such generic scale is the Quality of Life Profile (QLP) (Raphael et al., 1999). This was developed following an extensive review of available literature on quality of life and by undertaking qualitative research into QoL in people with and without learning or developmental disabilities.

The QLP allows for the assessment of the following domains: being, belonging and becoming; these domains are divided into three sub-domains (see Table 5.1). People are asked to rate both their enjoyment and the importance of the items listed in the profile on a five-point scale. With one indicating least and five indicating most, this means that an item can score highly on enjoyment but not on importance and vice versa. The domains identified in the QLP were the same as the themes identified in the Growing Older (GO) Programme (Walker, 2005) as being important to QoL. The GO programme was the largest social science investigation into ageing and older people undertaken in the UK. Table 5.1 relates the QLP to your practice by relating the profile to Frazer, one of the case scenarios you are following in this book (see website: **www.learningmatters.co.uk/nursing** for full case study).

Domain	Sub-domain	Items included in domain and sub-domain	Areas to consider
Being: concerned with who a person is	Physical	• Physical health • Personal hygiene • Nutrition • Exercise • Grooming and clothing • General physical appearance	Frazer has an ulcer on his foot which has become infected; this has resulted in reduced mobility, and though he is still able to move around he has to rest regularly.
	Psychological	• Psychological health and adjustment • Cognition • Feelings • Self-esteem and self-control	Frazer has not always managed his diabetes well; this has resulted in health complications. Frazer may have feelings of low self-esteem due to this as he realises the impact his diabetes may have on his life.
	Spiritual	• Personal values • Personal standards of conduct • Spiritual beliefs	By taking a more active role in his health management through action planning Frazer is maintaining hope for his future.

continued opposite...

continued...

Belonging: the connections a person has with their environment	Physical	• Home • Workplace/school • Neighbourhood • Community	Frazer is fully mobile and is able to travel around his local area, though due to an infection this is reduced at the moment.
	Social	• Intimate others • Family • Friends • Work colleagues • Neighbourhood and community	Frazer is married and has a daughter, Fiona, for whom he is the main carer. He works part time on account of this.
	Community	• Adequate income • Health and social services • Employment • Education programmes • Recreation programmes • Community events and activities	Both Frazer and his wife are working; Fiona is at primary school. Frazer is able to access his local health services: he regularly sees his practice nurse.
Becoming: achieving goals, hopes and aspirations	Practical	• Domestic activities • Employment • School or volunteer activities • Seeing to health and social needs	Frazer is able to help with the domestic activities and works part time to enable him to look after Fiona.
	Leisure	• Activities that promote relaxation and reduce stress	Frazer enjoys swimming and regularly takes Fiona with him, though due to his recent infection he has not been swimming as often.
	Growth	• Activities that promote maintenance or improvement of knowledge and skills • Adapting to change	Recently Frazer has taken a more active role in self-managing his diabetes: he has implemented an action plan to monitor his feet.

Table 5.1: Application of Raphael et al.'s (1999) QLP to your clinical practice

As you can see from Table 5.1, the QLP takes into account all aspects of a person, the QoL domains and how they are interrelated, e.g. Frazer's infection has an impact on aspects of his being, belonging and becoming. By assessing a person's QoL holistically the impact a change in their LTC has on their QoL can be seen. Understanding this will enable you to work with Frazer to put in place a plan of care that will reduce the impact his infection has on his QoL, resulting in an improved QoL. As well as affecting Frazer's QoL, his altering health status will affect the QoL of other family members. While for Frazer and his family this impact might be quite minimal, for other carers caring for a person with an LTC can severely impact on their QoL.

Research summary: Carer quality of life

As mentioned in Chapter 2, carers play a crucial role in the care and management of people living with LTCs. It is known that caring impacts on many areas of a carer's life and can result in increased physical strain, increased responsibility, and a decline in their mental health and social participation (Cohen et al., 2006). Cohen et al.'s (2006) quantitative study focused on QoL of carers caring for people with a life threatening illness (cancer). Their research focused on carer QoL in relation to different areas including in relation to the patient's condition. Their results concluded that the areas that impacted most negatively on a carer's QoL were 'patient condition' and 'carer's own state'. These findings support both Brewin's (2004) phenomenological study (lung disease) and Barnes et al.'s qualitative and quantitative study (2006) (heart failure).

Both Brewin (2004) and Barnes et al. (2006) used semistructured interviews. Carers were asked about their role as a carer, whether they had support and the effect of caring on their health and finances. Like Cohen et al. (2006), Brewin's (2004) results found that the carers carried an emotional burden regarding being a carer and expressed feelings of anger and frustration which impacted negatively on their QoL. Barnes et al. (2006) explicitly looked at carer health and found that carers who had a health condition themselves were at an increased risk of experiencing depression as a carer and experiencing a reduced QoL. However, Brewin (2004) noted that carers felt pride in their role and used humour to help them cope. She also noted that they felt socially isolated; however, like Cohen et al. (2006) she found that family support was beneficial to their QoL. In addition, Brewin stated that financial uncertainty and the lack of clarity over what was available impacted negatively on carer QoL, though for those working this did provide them with an outside interest which positively impacted on their QoL.

It is important to recognise the factors that impact on carer QoL. Measuring the QoL of carers will enable you to work with the carer to provide support and assistance to allow them to continue in their role as carer, improving not only their QoL but also the QoL of the person they are caring for.

Activity 5.2 *Decision-making*

Read over the following scenario.

Mary is 78; she lives with her husband in a two-storey house. She has two children, a son and a daughter and three grandchildren, and both children live locally and usually visit once a week. She has many friends that she sees on a regular basis and is an active member of the local community, delivering meals on wheels for the WRVS. When she has time she likes to help out with her grandchildren and often has them over to stay. Mary has no strong religious beliefs, though she has a strong moral code and is known as being pragmatic.

continued opposite...

continued...

Over the past few months she has been experiencing increasing shortness of breath, especially on exertion. As a keen golfer her dyspnoea has not been welcome; recently she had to stop golfing. As well as her shortness of breath she has been losing weight, her appetite has reduced as she occasionally finds eating painful and is experiencing dysphagia. She is able to take care of her hygiene needs and is still mobile, but has to walk slowly and can really only manage very short distances.

During the last six months Mary has undergone a series of investigations – chest x-ray, spirometry, blood tests and endoscopy – all of which were inconclusive. She has currently been given a diagnosis of COPD. However, due to her weight loss she recently had a CT scan, the results of which give a confirmed diagnosis of lung cancer (adenocarcinoma) with metastatic spread to her liver. Mary has been offered a course of chemotherapy to reduce tumour size and limit disease progression.

Using the information on QoL and Table 5.1 relate the QLP to the above scenario and answer the following questions.

- What is affecting Mary's QoL?
- Which areas of her life are being affected?

A brief outline answer is given at the end of the chapter.

As you will see from Activity 5.2, Mary's diagnosis has had a negative impact on many of the areas that influence her QoL. However, there are some areas that will impact positively, such as her strong family and social support. In Mary's situation you could use your assessment of her QoL to address some of the priorities of her care; for example, psychological support to help Mary and her family to come to terms with her diagnosis. Using information in Chapter 1 (the impact of being diagnosed with an LTC), Chapter 2 (emotional support) and Chapter 7 (breaking bad news) will assist you to do this.

The aim of effective symptom management is to provide a plan of care to reduce the symptoms a person is experiencing which would result in an increase in the person's QoL.

Symptom management in LTCs

Activity 5.1 (page 88) has shown you that people living with an LTC will experience many symptoms depending on the LTC they are living with. Effective symptom management requires an appropriate person-centred plan of care to be in place that addresses these symptoms. There are many ways that you can put together a plan of care for a person. Traditional care plans may be either pre-printed or hand written, core or individualised and may include care pathways. Working in collaboration with the person allows a personalised care plan to be drawn up. This has the benefit of ensuring that the care and management planned clearly meets their individual needs. Rather than achieving a 'best fit' for the person and their needs you achieve a 'perfect fit'. As they are time-consuming to write, however, a compromise may be to use core care plans that are personalised to the individual person and their needs (Barrett et al., 2009).

For people living with an LTC one of the most common therapeutic interventions used in symptom management is the use of medicines. It is relevant therefore that you have an understanding of the role that medicines management has in relation to the care and management of LTCs.

Medicines management

This is a crucial part of the care and management of LTCs as the use of medicines is the most common therapeutic intervention in the NHS (Carrier, 2009). However, it is known that up to 50% of people living with an LTC do not take their medication as prescribed. This has the potential to impact negatively on their health, quality of life and life expectancy. It can also increase healthcare costs. It is important that you understand how people living with LTCs view their medication if you are to support them in making good use of their prescribed medication (NPC, 2007a). The terms **concordance** and **compliance** are often used in medicines management. It is likely that if a medication regime has been reached concordantly it will be followed. However, this is not always the case. For example a person may be concordant with their medication regime but non-compliant because they are unable to open the blister pack in which their medication is dispensed (NPC, 2007a). In addition to such practical aspects factors such as a lack of information about the medication and what it does can have an impact. For example, a person with Parkinson's disease not appreciating the importance of taking their medication at the prescribed time may result in an increase in 'on/off' moments. Successful medicines management involves both concordance and compliance. Providing the person with relevant information regarding their medication, e.g. how the medication works and its effect on their symptoms and ensuring their medication is supplied in a suitable way, can contribute towards effective medicines management. One strategy that has been introduced to promote medicines management is the medicines use review.

The role of the pharmacist in medicines management in promoting self-management

Since 2005, in England, accredited community pharmacists have been able to undertake medicines use reviews (MURs). Similar medication services are available in Northern Ireland, Scotland and Wales. An MUR gives a person living with an LTC the opportunity to talk to their pharmacist about the medication they are taking. People can refer themselves for a MUR, they can be referred by members of the primary healthcare team or they may be selected by their GP. It should be noted that a person must have received their repeat prescription for at least three months before they are able to access a MUR with the pharmacist. The aim of an MUR is to (NPC, 2007b):

- support the person to learn more about their medicines, what they are for, how they work and how to take them for maximum benefit;
- identify any problems that the person may be having, e.g. side-effects, reading labels or ordering their medication;
- ensure that the most effective formulation is being prescribed, e.g. tablets, liquid;
- support the cost-effective use of medications and to encourage people not to stockpile medication or to over-order their medication.

Working with the person in this way increases their knowledge and understanding of their medication regime, increasing their concordance. It also impacts on their ability to self-manage their condition as correctly taking their medication means that they are receiving the maximum efficacy of the medication, reducing symptoms.

With a focus on pain management and nutrition and through the use of case scenarios and the nursing process the following section will develop your knowledge and skills in relation to symptom management in LTCs.

The nursing process and symptom management in LTCs

Holistic symptom management involves recognising the relationship between a person's physical, social, psychological and spiritual health and the impact this has on their symptoms and how they manage them. As a nurse involved in the care and management of people living with an LTC, using the nursing process (Yura and Walsh, 1973) enables you to work with the person, their family and carers, to successfully manage their symptoms. Whether you use Roper, Logan and Tierney's activities of daily living model (Roper et al., 2000), Orem's self-care model (1980) or the tidal model (Barker, 2001), as your nursing model, the nursing process is the means by which you implement your model. The nursing process is a four-step process – assess, plan, implement and evaluate – and is inherent within the *Standards for Pre-registration Nursing Education* (Nursing and Midwifery Council, 2010). Over the years this process has been adapted and refined: Barrett et al. (2009) have included a further two steps to the nursing process to aid problem solving:

- assess;
- systematic nursing diagnosis;
- plan;
- implement;
- recheck;
- evaluate.

This six-step process can be remembered by the acronym ASPIRE. When using the nursing process it is important to remember that all steps are interrelated. A plan cannot be made unless an assessment has taken place and a systematic nursing diagnosis has been made; care cannot be evaluated unless a plan has been implemented and rechecked. For the nursing process to be used effectively you must possess effective communication skills, have developed a positive therapeutic relationship, have a sound knowledge of the LTC the person is living with and how the symptoms of this can be managed. Used efficiently and in partnership with the person living with an LTC, the nursing process can ensure holistic symptom management.

The management of pain in LTCs

Pain is *an unpleasant sensory and emotional experience associated with actual or potential tissue damage* (International Association for the Study of Pain, 1986).

The perception of pain evolved in humans to warn us of danger so we can take action to avoid damage. For example, we withdraw our hand from a flame to avoid getting burnt. However, for people with an LTC it is not possible to withdraw from the pain as the pain may be caused by the condition. To help you to provide effective pain management to people with LTCs it is important to have an understanding of the mechanisms of how we feel pain and the different types of pain. To support you to do this answer the following questions:

- How do we feel pain?
- What is the difference between nociceptive and neuropathic pain?
- What are the body's natural analgesics?

A brief outline answer is given at the end of the chapter.

As you can see from Activity 5.3, there are differences in the way pain is experienced, whether it is acute and chronic, and in how the pain is transmitted via the nervous system. It is therefore important to know if the person is experiencing acute or chronic pain and whether it is nociceptive or neuropathic, as this will influence the management of the pain. However, it should be noted that pain is not purely a series of physiological processes.

Pain is what the patient says it is.

(Thomas, 2003, page 124)

Pain is experienced by people and families – not nerve endings.

(Dame Cicely Saunders)

Pain is a common symptom for people living with an LTC and for many people it is their major concern. For many their pain will be chronic: the Chronic Pain Policy Coalition (CPPC) aims to have pain recognised as the fifth vital sign (CPPC, 2007). Through early assessment and treatment their aim is to improve the QoL of people living with an LTC who are experiencing chronic pain. Pain has many causes and means different things to different people: it changes during the course of an LTC and its treatment and management vary from person to person (Endacott et al., 2009). This highlights the individual nature of pain. In the 1960s, as a result of her research with terminally ill people Dame Cicely Saunders developed the concept of 'total pain'. 'Total pain' incorporates the physical, social, spiritual and psychological aspects of a person; these aspects then interact to produce a person's individual pain experience (Clark, 2002). Table 5.2 outlines some of the factors that can influence a person's 'total pain' as applied to Mary (see Activity 5.2).

Aspects	Influencing factors	Application to practice
Physical	The condition The person's functional capacity Side-effects of treatment Disfigurement	Mary's underlying lung cancer is causing her pain when she swallows, and this may affect her nutritional intake and have a knock-on effect on her health. As yet she has not commenced treatment but she is due to undergo a course of chemotherapy which may result in increased fatigue and muscle tiredness
Social	Family issues Loss of role at work Loss of role at home Finances Change in appearance due to condition Sense of helplessness	Mary is experiencing a loss of her role as mother and grandmother. She has had to stop playing golf and may soon have to stop helping with meals on wheels
Spiritual	Purpose Religion Meaning Uncertainty about future Hope Fear of pain/death	Due to having to stop some of her social activities, Mary may feel a loss of purpose. Her diagnosis may have prompted feelings of uncertainty and fear, though she may also experience feelings of hope as she commences her treatment
Psychological	Anger Delays in diagnosis Coping ability Control and sense of usefulness Failure of treatment	Due to the delay in diagnosis Mary may be experiencing anger and resentment and asking 'what if?' Her pragmatic nature may help her to focus on practical aspects and increase her sense of control and usefulness

Table 5.2: 'Total pain': aspects, influencing factors and application to practice

This personal construct of pain means that pain is subjective, making an unbiased objective assessment of it complex and challenging. You must remain objective at all times and recognise how your perceptions and the individuality of the person can impact on pain perception. If you use the nursing process to structure your care and management of a person's pain, then undertaking a comprehensive assessment of a person and their pain is the first step to successful management.

Assessing pain in long term conditions

Activity 5.4   *Evidence-based practice and research*

Case study: Angela

It is 11 years since Angela's diagnosis of RRMS. During this time she has given birth to her second son Jack, now aged nine; her oldest son Charlie is 11. Over the past 11 years Angela has experienced several relapses of her MS, with two affecting her right leg. Angela's last relapse eight weeks ago has left her with residual spasms in her leg, causing musculoskeletal pain and discomfort. Angela now works part time as a librarian and her husband James is still working as a software engineer for a defence company, though recent promotion has meant he has been away from home quite a lot.

Angela is at home, though she is still off work. You are spending time with the MS clinical nurse specialist (CNS) who is visiting Angela following her recent relapse. During this consultation Angela mentions her residual spasms and musculoskeletal pain. Angela's pain is due to muscle spasm, caused by increased muscle tone due to nerve damage, causing the stretch muscles in her lower leg to become hyperactive. Her spasms and associated musculoskeletal pain are worse at night; she has been using the relaxation techniques that she has used previously. However, she is still experiencing pain.

Reflecting back on the concept of 'total pain', what could be contributing to Angela's pain and what methods could you and the CNS use to assess Angela's 'total pain'?

A brief outline answer is given at the end of the chapter.

Activity 5.4 has demonstrated that there are many ways in which a person's pain can be assessed. It may be that you may have to try more than one method of assessment until you find one that is suitable. Consistency of pain assessment is important to enable a clear picture of a person's pain to be obtained. Therefore it is important that the same method of pain assessment is used each time a person's pain is assessed. For some people, e.g., those with cognitive impairment or a learning disability, ensuring effective pain assessment can be challenging and may result in pain being undiagnosed or undertreated.

Pain assessment in cognitive impairment

Undiagnosed or under treated pain in people with cognitive impairment may be due to a variety of reasons. In Alzheimer's disease, for example, many of the areas of the brain that are affected, the hippocampus and the prefrontal cortex, are also involved in processing pain (Porth and Matfin, 2010). People with cognitive impairment may underreport their pain because they have forgotten they were in pain, leading to the undertreatment (Scherder and Van Manen, 2005). However, people with cognitive impairment can experience the same physical health conditions as those without cognitive impairment (e.g., diabetes, COPD, musculoskeletal problems), and therefore it is likely that they experience similar amounts of pain as people without cognitive impairment.

continued opposite...

continued...

Many pain assessment tools require the person to verbalise their pain, which people with a cognitive impairment find difficult. Therefore as well as using picture scale tools, using specific pain assessment tools for people with cognitive impairment is important.

- Abbey pain scale – this is an assessment tool for use with people who have dementia and are not able to verbalise. Assessment is undertaken by observing the person and reporting on a variety of indicators. These include behaviour changes, e.g., increasing confusion, facial expressions, e.g., looking frightened and physical changes, e.g., contractures.
- Pain assessment in advanced dementia (PAINAD) – an observational tool that looks at the person's breathing, vocalising, facial expression, body language and how consolable they are.
- The disability distress assessment tool – this is used to help identify distress cues in people with cognitive impairment or limited communication. It describes the person's normal behaviour; for example, what vocal sounds they make when they are content and what sounds they make when they are distressed. A note is then made of what situations are known to cause the person distress. Once completed, this assessment tool can be used to identify times when a person is distressed. While this tool identifies distress it can be a useful indicator of pain.

Working with the person's carer, especially to find out what the person's normal behaviour is, will enhance any pain assessment carried out. This section reiterates that it is the process of assessment and the knowledge and skills you use and not just the assessment tool being used that is important (Endacott et al., 2009).

Having used a holistic approach to assessing Angela's pain, alongside an appropriate pain assessment tool, you are now able to work with Angela to plan and implement an effective plan of care.

Planning and implementing pain management in LTCs

In implementing a plan of care to manage a person's pain it is important to realise that there are many methods that can be used to manage pain in LTCs. These range from medication, both prescribed and over-the-counter, the use of physiotherapy and psychological care. The methods used will differ depending on the person and the type of pain being experienced. In the case of musculoskeletal pain, the management may focus on physiotherapy, relaxation and medication. The management of neuropathic pain may consist of physiotherapy, for advice regarding posture and positioning, the use of antidepressant and anticonvulsant medication and relaxation (Gray, 2004). It may not be possible to achieve complete pain relief for everyone; if this is the case, the aim will be to reduce the pain to a level that is tolerable for the person.

Case study: Angela

Angela's pain assessment had revealed that she was experiencing musculoskeletal pain radiating down her right calf and into her foot on six nights out of seven and occasionally during the day on four out of seven days. Angela scored her pain as being seven out of ten and described it as 'aching'; she was aware this was disturbing her usual sleep pattern and was concerned that this would increase her fatigue. The aim of the plan of care agreed between Angela and her MS CNS was to reduce both the frequency (to three out of five nights and two out of seven days) and intensity (to four) of Angela's pain as well as to improve the quality of her sleep. Following consultation they agreed a plan of care, as follows.

Physiotherapy

The MS CNS will refer Angela to the community physiotherapist for an assessment and a planned programme of stretching exercises to help lengthen Angela's calf muscles to reduce spasm and spasticity. Physiotherapy has been shown to reduce the use of analgesics in people with MS (Gray, 2004). These exercises will need to be carried out on a daily basis and Angela has agreed to write up an action plan (see Chapter 4) to ensure she is able to do this. The MS CNS has also asked that the physiotherapist consider using transcutaneous electrical nerve stimulation (TENS) as a non-pharmacological means of managing Angela's pain. The evidence surrounding TENS is varied; however it is used in the management of pain in a variety of situations. TENS stimulates the nervous system through the use of transcutaneous electrodes; this stimulation is thought to reduce the transmission of pain signals to the brain, altering the person's perception of their pain.

Prescribed medication

As a qualified nurse/independent prescriber Angela's MS CNS is able to prescribe any licensed medication, within the sphere of her clinical competence (NPC, 2010). Based on her assessment of Angela and her pain she has prescribed an initial dose of Baclofen: 5 mg, three times a day. This can be gradually increased depending on the degree of relief Angela is experiencing. By reducing the transmission of electrical impulse along the nerves in Angela's central nervous system Baclofen will cause Angela's muscles to relax, reducing the amount of spasm and pain. As well as outlining to Angela how Baclofen works, the MS CNS has provided Angela with information regarding some of the common side-effects:

- *gastrointestinal upset: Angela has been advised to take her Baclofen after eating food and in case of nausea to eat little and often;*
- *dry mouth: chewing sugar-free gum or sweets can help reduce Angela's dry mouth;*
- *drowsiness: before driving Angela should make sure her reaction time is normal – alcohol should be avoided as it may increase her drowsiness;*
- *dizziness: getting up from either lying or sitting slowly – if the feeling continues Angela could lie down for a few minutes until the dizziness passes.*

The MS CNS has also advised Angela that if she is concerned regarding any aspect of this medication to contact her and not to stop taking it suddenly as sudden withdrawal can cause severe side-effects. The MS CNS will visit Angela weekly over the next six weeks to review the benefits of the treatment.

continued opposite...

continued...

Over-the-counter medication

As well as taking her prescribed medication Angela may also be taking over-the-counter medication to help manage her pain, e.g., paracetamol or ibuprofen. If this is the case it is important that the MS CNS identifies this as it is known that ibuprofen reduces the rate at which Baclofen is excreted from the body, resulting in an increased risk of toxicity (British National Formulary, 2010). Therefore Angela should be advised to use paracetamol in preference to ibuprofen.

Relaxation

Angela has decided to continue with her relaxation techniques, especially at night. While this does not reduce her spasm and associated musculoskeletal pain it does help reduce her levels of stress and improves the quality of her sleep (Lorig et al., 2006). Improving the quality of Angela's sleep will reduce the likelihood of her experiencing increasing fatigue.

Both Angela and the MS CNS agreed that Angela should continue to assess her musculoskeletal pain on a regular basis and devise her own action plan (Chapter 4) to identify when and how this will be done. The effectiveness of the above plan of care will be rechecked against Angela's initial pain assessment and her ongoing assessment of her musculoskeletal pain. This recheck will allow specific information, such as Angela's assessment of her pain, to be linked to the plan of care that was implemented. In the initial stages this recheck will be done on a weekly basis for the next four weeks, providing ongoing support for Angela. A formal evaluation would take place at the end of four weeks.

It was decided not to refer Angela to an occupational therapist regarding splinting at this stage but to evaluate the above plan of care and refer if there was no improvement in Angela's spasm and pain.

As you can see Angela and her MS CNS worked collaboratively to compile the above plan of care. Empowerment was maintained by incorporating action planning, enabling Angela to fit her physiotherapy and pain assessment into her daily routine. By recognising the benefits Angela experiences in relation to her relaxation, though this does not directly improve her pain, will positively reflect on her QoL. The role of the MS CNS was to provide specialist knowledge regarding the pharmacological management of Angela's spasm and associated musculoskeletal pain and to refer to other members of the multidisciplinary team to maximise Angela's pain relief.

Evaluating pain management in LTCs

Evaluating the care implemented is the final stage of the nursing process: the process of evaluation allows you to understand whether the care implemented has been successful in meeting the person's identified needs. Evaluating the care implemented requires a collaborative approach and should be based on how well the aims of the care implemented have been met. Evaluating care requires you to be able to analyse all stages of the nursing process, e.g., was the pain assessment tool used appropriate, was the stated aim achievable and were the planned interventions suitable for the person and their needs (Barrett et al., 2009)? By breaking the process down into its component parts, you are able to evaluate which parts were successful and which parts were not. Evaluating your care and management in this way allows you to reflect on your practice, prompting both personal and professional development.

Case study: Angela

Four weeks after your initial visit to Angela with her MS CNS both you and the MS CNS are visiting Angela to evaluate the plan of care that was implemented. Angela has continued to assess her pain as outlined in her action plan; she is now experiencing pain on four nights out of seven and on two days out of seven, with her pain intensity having reduced to between three and four. She also reports that while she is still experiencing pain on four nights out of seven the quality of her sleep has improved.

Physiotherapy
Angela has found the physiotherapy to be very beneficial and has worked hard to ensure she carries out her exercises every day. As well as exercising her right leg she has been doing the same exercises with her left leg and has noticed a reduction in the severity of the muscle spasms. Angela feels this has contributed the most in reducing her musculoskeletal pain. She has not had any TENS yet, though this has been recommended by the physiotherapist.

Prescribed medication
Angela continues to take 5 mg of Baclofen three times a day; she did experience some side-effects when she initially started taking the Baclofen, mainly nausea and some dizziness. However, she is able to manage these. Despite still experiencing pain on four out of seven nights she is not keen to increase her dose of Baclofen yet.

Over-the-counter medication
Angela has not been taking any regular over-the-counter analgesics.

Relaxation
Angela finds this really beneficial, especially in managing with her levels of stress and improving the quality of her sleep. Despite being awake due to her pain she is able to remain calm and relaxed, increasing the chances of her being able to get back to sleep.

Following the evaluation of the care implemented against the original aims of the care, both Angela and her MS CNS note that while the severity of Angela's pain has reduced and the quality of her sleep has improved she is still experiencing pain on four nights out of seven. As Angela is not keen to increase the dose of her Baclofen her MS CNS suggests that she asks her physiotherapist about using TENS at night. Angela agrees to this suggestion and will discuss it with her physiotherapist at her next appointment. A further recheck meeting is planned for one week's time.

In this case study the aims of the initial plan of care were not fully met, demonstrating the cyclical nature of the nursing process. During the process of evaluation not only do you evaluate the care that has been delivered to date, you also undertake an assessment of the person's new baseline. This then leads into the planning, implementation and evaluation of further interventions.

Activity 5.5   *Decision-making*

Case study: Andrew

Andrew's level of exercise has increased since he implemented his action plan. He still experiences dyspnoea but is able to manage this more effectively. Andrew has noticed that his clothes seem a bit large and is concerned he might be losing weight. You are visiting Andrew with his district nurse when he brings this up. When assessing Andrew using the malnutrition universal screening tool (British Association for Enteral and Parenteral Nutrition (BAPEN), 2003) it is noted that his body mass index (BMI) is 20 (poor protein energy status possible) giving him a score of 1, his weight loss of less than 5% gives him a score of 0 resulting in an overall score of 1. This places Andrew at medium risk: the MUST management guidelines state that Andrew's dietary intake should be recorded for three days and reviewed. Andrew's district nurse asks him to keep a food diary for the next three days and arranges another appointment to visit on the fourth day.

On your return visit it is evident from Andrew's food diary that he is not consuming an adequate and balanced nutritional intake. This is important, as a reduced nutritional intake could result in worsening of his respiratory muscle function and increase his dyspnoea and the likelihood of him developing further chest infections (BAPEN, 2003).

What plan of care would you implement to address Andrew's poor nutritional intake and what members of the multidisciplinary team would you involve?

Useful advice is available on the use of MUST and care planning via the BAPEN website at **www.bapen.org.uk/musttoolkit.html**.

A brief outline answer is given at the end of the chapter.

As you will have seen from Activity 5.5, many of the symptoms experienced by people living with an LTC are interrelated, with one symptom having an effect on other aspects of the person's health and wellbeing. Having an understanding of the common signs and symptoms of specific LTCs and how they are managed will assist you in your delivery of appropriate and effective symptom management.

Conclusion

Having read through this chapter and worked through the activities, you will have developed your knowledge and skills in relation to symptom management in the care and management of people living with an LTC. How you use this new knowledge and skills will depend on where you are working and your roles and responsibilities. However, as a nurse you can improve the care you provide to people living with an LTC, and their carers, by recognising the importance of maintaining QoL and the factors that influence QoL. By using the being, belonging and becoming model you will be able to provide holistic symptom management for those in your care. Using the nursing process, to work collaboratively with those living with an LTC, will ensure that the care and management you provide is based on a good assessment of the person's needs and is clearly focused on addressing those needs. It will also encourage you to reflect on your practice, further developing your knowledge and skills in relation to many aspects of person-centred care.

Chapter summary

This chapter has provided you with an overview of QoL in people living with an LTC and the role that effective symptom management has in promoting and enhancing QoL. It has outlined the importance of concordance and compliance in relation to medicines management and how the medicines use review can assist in achieving this. By relating the nursing process to symptom management it has emphasised the importance of person-centred care in the effective management of symptoms in people living with an LTC.

Activities: brief outline answers

Activity 5.1: Evidence-based practice and research (page 88)

Coronary heart disease (CHD)

Coronary heart disease is the main cause of angina pectoris and the main symptom of angina pectoris is pain. Pain is felt in the chest and can feel, tight, heavy or dull. Pain can radiate to the left arm, jaw, neck and back. Other symptoms that may be present are breathlessness, nausea, fatigue and dizziness. It is important to find out what the pain is like (location, severity, character and duration), what they were doing before the pain started (level of exertion, emotional state, eating a large meal or in cold weather) and how stable their symptoms are (is the pain predictable?) (Clinical Knowledge Summaries (CKS), 2009c).

In CHD atherosclerotic plaques in the coronary arteries cause progressive narrowing of the lumen of the arteries. This narrowing results in reduced blood flow to the myocardium, especially during times when extra demand is being made, e.g. during exercise. There are a number of known causes of CHD; these include smoking, hypertension, high cholesterol and diabetes (Porth and Matfin, 2010). To effectively manage the symptoms of the disease, these causes should be addressed. Advice should be given regarding smoking cessation, reducing the amount of saturated fat and increasing the amount of fish and fruit and vegetables in their diet can help reduce their cholesterol, as can taking regular exercise. It is important to ensure that any prescribed medication, (e.g., statins, beta-blockers) are taken as prescribed (CKS, 2009c).

Rheumatoid arthritis (RA)

This is a chronic auto-immune disease, which affects the small joints of the hands and feet, though other joints can be involved. As the disease progresses any system of the body can be affected by the underlying inflammatory processes. The main symptoms of RA are pain and swelling in the joints of the hands and feet; the pain is usually worse at rest or during periods of inactivity. Stiffness and loss of function is also present. Stiffness is common in the morning and usually lasts more than 30 minutes. People can also experience fatigue, loss of weight and flu-like symptoms (CKS, 2009d).

In RA the synovium (membrane surrounding a joint that produces synovial fluid, which helps to keep the joint mobile) becomes swollen due to inflammatory processes. This process causes an increase in the production of synovial fluid into the joint, resulting in a swollen and painful joint. Over time the inflamed membrane causes joint erosion (Porth and Matfin, 2010). For people with RA, taking care of their joints is important in the management of symptoms, and ensuring a good balance between rest and exercise is crucial. It is known that inflamed joints should be rested; however, too much rest can cause joints to become stiff and weak due to muscle wasting. For the person with RA, recognising what activities increase pain and swelling and resting after this, or finding alternative ways of doing things, is relevant. Swimming is an excellent form of exercise as it is non-weight-bearing; exercise will also ensure a healthy weight is maintained, minimising stress on the joints (CKS, 2009d).

Medication management is an important aspect of the management of RA, therefore ensuring that the person is concordant with their medication regime is important. Disease-modifying anti-rheumatic drugs (DMARDs) taken in combination are the most effective way of managing symptoms and increasing quality of life (CKS, 2009d).

Parkinson's disease (PD)

This is a neurological disease that affects the substantia nigra in the brain. The substantia nigra produces dopamine, a neurotransmitter that assists in the transmission of motor nerve impulses to the muscles. Over time the cells in the substantia nigra die, causing a decline in the production of dopamine and associated reduction in the transmission of nervous impulses to the muscles (Porth and Matfin, 2010). This results in the following symptoms: bradykinesia – slow and shuffling gait; hypokinesia – difficulty with fine movements, e.g. buttoning clothes. A rest tremor may also be present, which may appear at the thumb and index finger (pin rolling) (CKS, 2009e). Other non-motor symptoms that may be present include falls, fatigue, constipation and sleep disturbance. It is important for individuals with PD to manage both the motor symptoms and the non-motor symptoms. Motor symptoms are managed by medication, e.g., Levodopa and dopamine agonists: these medications are dopamine substitutes and can improve motor function by increasing dopamine levels (CKS, 2009e). As with other LTCs, ensuring concordance with medication is important.

Due to postural instability, falls can be a common occurrence. The following can help address this: getting into a rhythm when walking, wearing appropriate footwear, taking medication correctly. If a person is constipated ensuring a diet high in fibre, fruit and vegetables, and drinking plenty of fluids, can help prevent constipation.

Activity 5.2: Decision-making (page 92)

Domain	Sub-domain	Items included in domain and sub-domain	Areas to consider
Being: concerned with who a person is	Physical	• Physical health • Personal hygiene • Nutrition • Exercise • Grooming and clothing • General physical appearance	Mary will no longer be able to take her regular exercise due to her dyspnoea. She is still able to take care of her personal hygiene though her nutritional intake is reduced due to her dysphagia.
	Psychological	• Psychological health and adjustment • Cognition • Feelings • Self-esteem and self-control	This is a devastating diagnosis for Mary and her family who will still be coming to terms with her diagnosis. This has the potential to negatively affect her psychologically, with feelings of disbelief, frustration, etc.
	Spiritual	• Personal values • Personal standards of conduct • Spiritual beliefs	At present Mary may not see any hope for the future; while she does not have any strong religious beliefs her personal beliefs will offer her support.

— continued overleaf...

Domain	Sub-domain	Items included in domain and sub-domain	Areas to consider
Belonging: the connections a person has with their environment	Physical	• Home • Work place/school • Neighbourhood • Community	Mary is still able to move around her house; however, her dyspnoea has compromised her ability to get out and about.
	Social	• Intimate others • Family • Friends • Work colleagues • Neighbourhood and community	Mary has a husband and close family, though she may realise that she is no longer able to look after her grandchildren overnight. Stopping golf may mean that she does not see friends as often.
	Community	• Adequate income • Health and social services • Employment • Education programmes • Recreation programmes • Community events and activities	Mary and her husband are both pensioners, and they may be eligible for some financial benefits. Mary is able to access relevant health services.
Becoming: achieving goals, hopes and aspirations	Practical	• Domestic activities • Employment • School or volunteer activities • Seeing to health and social needs	Due to her dyspnoea Mary may not be able to take care of her house and garden, increasing the work for her husband. She may also have to stop her WRVS meals on wheels work.
	Leisure	• Activities that promote relaxation and reduce stress	Mary is no longer able to play golf.
	Growth	• Activities that promote maintenance or improvement of knowledge and skills • Adapting to change	Mary may wish to learn ways to manage her dyspnoea and how to increase her nutritional intake. This approach may also help Mary and her family adapt to the changes.

As you can see from the above it is clear that Mary's dyspnoea and associated reduction in her mobility and ability to undertake her normal activities is having a major impact on her QoL. It is also evident that Mary's diagnosis is having a negative aspect on her QoL, affecting aspects of her being, belonging and becoming.

Activity 5.3: Critical thinking (page 96)

What are the body's natural analgesics?

The body's natural analgesics are opioid peptides (dynophorins and endorphins) produced in the hypothalamus and pituitary gland that are found in the nervous system in the areas of the brain associated with pain reception. They are also found in areas of the spinal cord. Their distribution corresponds to the areas of the brain where electrical stimulation can control pain, such as the thalamus. When a person experiences pain these opiod peptides are released at the point where the pain signal enters the spinal cord and at the synapses in the thalamus, hypothalamus and cerebral cortex (Porth and Matfin, 2010).

How do we feel pain?

There are pain receptors (nociceptors) within our skin, periosteum, arterial walls, joint surfaces and the lining of our cranium. Damage to these tissues stimulates local pain receptors, allowing pain to be easily localised and identified, for example a person with osteoarthritis who has pain in their knees. Pain receptors in other parts of the body, mainly the organs, are supplied by a larger, more diffuse arrangement of pain receptors. This may make locating pain more difficult as the pain can be experienced over a larger area. There are some organs in the body where there are almost no pain receptors, e.g. the liver parenchyma and the alveoli in the lungs. However, the liver capsule, the bronchi and parietal pleura are very sensitive to pain. Pain receptors are free nerve endings that are activated by stimuli such as pressure (mechanoreceptors), extremes of temperature (thermoreceptors) and chemical substances (chemoreceptors) (Porth and Matfin, 2010). Chronic pain is felt due to the fact that pain receptors do not adapt to sustained stimulation but keep on being activated and producing signals. This is because the body's natural analgesics need to be stimulated to remind the person to protect that area of their body to help manage the pain. Acute and chronic pain sensations are transmitted via sensory nerves to the thalamus and hypothalamus. Acute pain sensations are transmitted via larger A-delta fibres that are able to carry a larger number of impulses while chronic pain sensations are transmitted via smaller C fibres carrying a lower number of impulses (Porth and Matfin, 2010).

What is the difference between nociceptive and neuropathic pain?

Nociceptive pain is pain that is felt due to the activation of pain receptors (nociceptors). This type of pain is usually due to tissue damage, e.g. trauma, surgery or disease progression. It is often described as sharp, aching, crushing or throbbing. Neuropathic pain is felt when the nerve itself is damaged by compression or infiltration; the damaged nerve then sends signals to the rest of the nervous system. Due to damage to the sensory nerves the pain may be experienced in an area where there is numbness. Neuropathic pain is often described as burning, stabbing or like pins and needles (Porth and Matfin, 2010). An example of this is shingles (herpes zoster infection); this can cause peripheral neuropathic pain. This pain is often described as hot, burning, stalling, shooting or tingling.

Activity 5.4: Evidence-based practice and research (page 98)

Aspects	Influencing factors	Application to practice
Physical	The condition The person's functional capacity Side-effects of treatment Disfigurement	Angela will realise that this symptom may be permanent and that she may experience further deteriorations in her functional capacity. Her disturbed sleep may be a contributing factor
Social	Family issues Loss of role at work Loss of role at home Finances Change in appearance due to condition Sense of helplessness	Angela is currently off work; depending on her illness benefits this may have a financial impact on her and her family.
Spiritual	Purpose Religion Meaning Uncertainty about future Hope Fear of pain/death	This relapse may be a reminder to Angela of the ongoing nature of her RRMS. She may be worried about future relapses and any residual deficit

continued overleaf...

continued...

Aspects	Influencing factors	Application to practice
Psychological	Anger Delays in diagnosis Coping ability Control and sense of usefulness Failure of treatment	Angela has successfully used relaxation in the past to manage symptoms such as anxiety; she can use them again here.

Some methods of pain assessment:

- taking a pain history – assessing the site, nature and duration of the pain as well as factors that relieve and exacerbate it;
- physical examination – may help confirm the cause of the pain; will also allow examination of other aspects, such as nutrition;
- body charts – pictures of the human body where the person can indicate and record the location of any pain; these can be updated;
- numerical and visual analogue scales – includes 0–3 and 0–10 numerical scale and the no pain to worse pain or no pain relief to complete pain relief visual analogue scale;
- picture scales – use of faces with expressions ranging from happiness to distress;
- pain questionnaires and inventories – these question the person on a range of factors relating to their pain, e.g., pain intensity, mood, pain relief.

Using communication skills, such as active listening, touch, and observation and engaging in a therapeutic relationship with Angela, will enhance the assessment process, enabling you and Angela to work together to manage her pain.

Activity 5.5: Decision-making (page 103)

The aim of your plan of care would be to increase both the nutritional value and the quantity of food Andrew is eating. You would want to recheck the progress and appropriateness of your plan of care weekly with a formal evaluation being arranged in approximately four weeks' time. In order to implement a plan of care that reflects Andrew's needs it may be appropriate to ask some of the following questions.

- What local shops are there for Andrew to shop in?
- How does he get there; does he need transport?
- Is Andrew interested in food and meal preparation?
- Does his dyspnoea prevent him from preparing a meal?
- What is his regular eating pattern and preferences?

What is a healthy diet?
Provide Andrew with information regarding what is a healthy diet and the importance of including vitamins, minerals, fibre, protein, carbohydrate and fat. Due to the possibility of Andrew's diet being protein-poor, providing him with food choices and meals that will increase his protein intake is important, e.g., meat, fish, eggs and milk. Increasing the amount of protein in Andrew's diet will improve his immune system and help his body to repair any damaged tissue.

Access to healthy food
Depending on what access to shops Andrew has it may be necessary to arrange transport to take him to a shop where there is more access to fresh fruit and other foods. Alternatively, if Andrew has internet access he could order his shopping on line and have it delivered to his flat. Andrew may find this convenient as he can then conserve his energy for food preparation rather than shopping.

Eating and dyspnoea

Suggesting that Andrew has smaller but more frequent meals that are high in calories, and that he starts his meal with the calorie-high foods, may help him meet his energy requirements more efficiently. Avoiding carbonated drinks and foods such as beans and cabbage can reducing bloating and ease breathing.

It may be appropriate to refer Andrew to a dietician for further advice and support regarding his diet.

Further reading

Barrett, D, Wilson, B and Woollands, A (2009) *Care Planning: A Guide for Nurses.* Harlow: Pearson Education Limited.
This has a useful chapter on the nursing process, and contains other relevant information in relation to care planning.

Kerr, D, Cunningham, C and Wilkinson, H (2006) *Responding to the Pain Experiences of People with a Learning Difficulty and Dementia.* York: Joseph Rowntree Foundation.
An interesting and useful resource discussing pain in people with a learning disability who also have dementia.

Latter, S. (2010) Evidence base for effective medicines management. *Nursing Standard,* 24 (43): 62–66.
An article aimed at raising the awareness of nurse prescribers of the factors that influence a person's concordance and compliance with their medication.

Useful websites

www.npc.co.uk
The home page of the National Prescribing Centre; contains useful information regarding all areas of prescribing, including non-medical prescribing.

Chapter 6
Managing complex care in long term conditions

NMC Standards for Pre-registration Nursing Education

This chapter will address the following competencies:

Domain 1: Professional values

6. All nurses must understand the roles and responsibilities of other health and social care professionals, and seek to work with them collaboratively for the benefit of all who need care.

8. All nurses must practise independently, recognising the limits of their competence and knowledge. They must reflect on these limits and seek advice from, or refer to, other professionals where necessary.

Domain 3: Nursing practice and decision-making

4. All nurses must ascertain and respond to the physical, social and psychological needs of people, groups and communities. They must then plan, deliver and evaluate safe, competent, person-centred care in partnership with them, paying special attention to changing health needs during different life stages, including progressive illness and death, loss and bereavement.

4.1 Adult nurses must safely use invasive and non-invasive procedures, medical devices, and current technological and pharmacological interventions, where relevant, in medical and surgical nursing practice, providing information and taking account of individual needs and preferences.

8.1 Adult nurses must work in partnership with people who have long term conditions that require medical or surgical nursing, and their families and carers, to provide therapeutic nursing interventions, optimise health and wellbeing, facilitate choice and maximise self-care and self-management.

NMC Essential Skills Clusters

This chapter will address the following ESCs:

Cluster: Organisational aspects of care

13. People can trust the newly registered graduate nurse to promote continuity when their care is to be transferred to another service or person.

By the second progression point:

1. Assists in preparing people and carers for transfer and transition through effective dialogue and accurate information.

continued opposite...

continued...

3. Assists in the preparation of records and reports to facilitate safe and effective transfer.

Cluster: Medicines management

40. People can trust the newly registered graduate nurse to work in partnership with people receiving medical treatments and their carers.

By the second progression point:

1. Under supervision involves people and carers in administration and self-administration of medicines.

By entry to the register:

2. Works with people and carers to provide clear and accurate information.

3. Assesses the person's ability to safely self-administer their medicines.

Chapter aims

After reading this chapter you will be able to:

- understand the role case management has in the management of people with LTCs who have complex care needs;
- explain the roles and responsibilities of the case manager in the care of people living with an LTC;
- use care pathways to support person-centred care for those living with an LTC who have complex needs;
- recognise the importance of effective discharge planning for people living with an LTC and their carers.

Introduction

Evidence shows that intensive, ongoing and personalised case management can improve the quality of life and outcomes for people with the most complex long term conditions. A case management approach anticipates, coordinates and joins up care, reflecting these peoples' intricate health and social care needs.

(DH, 2006c, page 3)

The majority of people living with an LTC will have their condition managed effectively through appropriate health promotion and health education, self-management and timely symptom management. However, some people living with one or more LTCs will have more complex health and social care needs. For example, they may be at risk of admission and subsequent readmission to hospital care. It is estimated that there are approximately 25 people in a typical general practice for whom case management would be advantageous (DH, 2005b). This group of people, for a variety of reasons, e.g. living with more than one LTC, multiple episodes of unplanned hospital admissions or living on their own, can be intensive users of services. As a result of their many health and social care needs they are likely to experience a reduced quality of life. They require integrated and proactive care and management, coordinated by a suitably qualified person.

> ### Case study: Andrew
>
> *Andrew is a 76-year-old widower and is living with chronic obstructive pulmonary disease (COPD). Andrew lives alone in a one-bedroomed flat in a sheltered housing complex.*
>
> *Over the last 12 months Andrew has been experiencing worsening health, and has had two admissions to hospital, for chest infections, in the last three months. This is despite his district nurse working with Andrew to increase his level of exercise and improve his nutritional intake. After some initial success Andrew was not able to maintain his level of exercise and due to his increasing dyspnoea he has been relying on meals on wheels to provide him with a hot meal. His recent chest infections have left him with worsening dyspnoea and associated reduction in his mobility. Care workers visit twice a day to assist Andrew with washing and dressing, and a neighbour pops in to dust, vacuum and help with his laundry. At the weekly practice meeting, following his last admission, his GP has transferred Andrew's care over to the community matron for case management.*
>
> *David will be Andrew's case manager; David is a qualified district nurse and, working as part of the practice team, will be responsible for coordinating Andrew's care and management. David will use a case management approach to ensure that Andrew's ongoing physical, social and psychological needs are met. By leading, and taking responsibility for, Andrew's care David will coordinate input from other agencies, ensuring that Andrew's care needs are met. Through working with Andrew, and as his single point of contact, David will support Andrew to make informed choices about the care he receives. David will further work with Andrew to encourage him to be aware of changes in his condition that signal an exacerbation and to take action to address these.*

Andrew's story demonstrates that the aim of case management is to streamline care and the management of complex needs that result from living with one or more LTCs. As a student nurse you may not be directly involved in the case management of people living with an LTC, though it may be that, when working with a community matron or specialist respiratory nurse, you observe the management of complex care needs for this group of people. Integrating the knowledge from previous chapters in relation to health promotion and health education, self-management and symptom management will enable you to assist in the delivery of effective case management and complex care. To further support you in your role this chapter will develop your knowledge and understanding of case management and complex care. In order to do this the chapter will discuss the roles and responsibilities of case managers and how complex care is managed. The chapter also discusses the way in which care pathways can be used in managing complex care and examines the importance of discharge planning for those living with an LTC who have been admitted to secondary care.

Policy review

Case management is an essential part of the care and management of people living with an LTC. It has been defined as being *the process of planning, co-ordinating, managing and reviewing the care of an individual*; here the goal is *to develop cost-effective and efficient ways of coordinating services in order to improve quality of life* (Hutt et al., 2004, page 6).

Although case management is only briefly mentioned in the *National Service Framework (NSF) for Long Term Conditions* (Department of Health (DH), 2005a), it forms a more integral part of other policy documents. In England it is embedded in the National Health Service (NHS) and Social Care Model (DH, 2005b), and forms part of the Kaiser Permanente service delivery model and is represented as the apex of the triangle (see page 11). The approach taken in Northern Ireland has been to focus on the delivery of effective primary care services, including those for people living with an LTC (Department of Health, Social Services and Public Safety, 2005). Objective 6 includes the development of case management to support those with complex care needs. In Scotland it forms part of high impact change 4, how services for people living with an LTC are delivered. Case management is used to provide care for those with complex needs, with the case manager responsible for coordinating the care (Scottish Government Health Delivery Directorate Improvement Support Team, 2009). In Wales, case management forms part of their integrated model, with the approach taken similar to that used in England, and is used to ensure that those with complex needs receive coordinated and responsive care (Department of Health and Social Services, 2007).

Case management in LTCs

Case management originated in the USA where, in the 1950s, it was used as a means of providing care to people with severe mental health needs. From this it was then rolled out and used with older people who had complex health and social care needs. Its aim was to increase coordination of services, to reduce healthcare costs and minimise the need for long term care (Drennan and Goodman, 2004). In the UK case management has been used in mental health nursing since the 1980s; this was as a response to the shift from institutionalised to community care. Its role in the care and management of people with mental health needs is recognised in the *NSF for Mental Health: Modern Standards and Service Models* (DH, 1999). Here it forms part of standards four and five: *Effective services for people with severe mental illness*. Since then, as mentioned in the policy section above, it has formed part of the care and management of people living with an LTC. The aim of case management is to provide the person living with an LTC with care and management that focuses on reducing and preventing unplanned admission to secondary care.

Activity 6.1   *Reflection*

Case management is a key part of the care and management of people living with an LTC. On your own or with a group of colleagues, reflect on the areas where you have undertaken clinical practice and consider the following questions.

- What members of the health and social care team undertake the role of case manager?
- What are their roles and responsibilities in relation to managing the care of people with LTCs?
- How do they fit in with other health and social care professionals?

As the answers will be based on your own observations there is no outline answer at the end of this chapter.

Undertaking Activity 6.1 will have shown you that case management can be undertaken by a range of health and social care professionals. These may include district nurses, nurse specialists and community matrons, physiotherapists and social workers. The DH has identified the following two levels of case management to be used in the care and management of LTCs (DH, 2005b).

- Case management and case managers – responsible for coordinating the care and management of people living with an LTC who have a complex single LTC or social need. They will be responsible for planning, monitoring and anticipating the needs of those living with one or more LTCs. In this situation the case manager is likely to be a qualified nurse, social worker or other healthcare professional.
- Case management and community matrons – in addition to the responsibilities outlined above for case managers, community matrons provide advanced clinical nursing skills, e.g., physical health assessment, non-medical prescribing and the management of acute exacerbations.

Whereas the level of clinical nursing care may vary between the levels of case management identified above, the roles and responsibilities of the case manager/community matron should be underpinned by the following core elements (Hutt et al., 2004):

- case finding or screening;
- assessment;
- care planning;
- implementation of care plan;
- monitoring and reviewing.

These core elements are explored in greater detail in the next section of this chapter where they are related to Andrew and his community matron David.

Roles and responsibilities of the case manager/ community matron in LTCs

It is the responsibility of the case manager/community matron to ensure that the core elements listed above form the basis of their roles and responsibilities in relation to people living with an LTC. Using Andrew's case scenario, Table 6.1 provides you with some points to consider and applies these core elements to clinical practice.

As you can see from Table 6.1, the core elements of case management allow David, as Andrew's community matron, to coordinate and guide his care. Ensuring a single point of contact will improve communication between all health and social care professionals involved in Andrew's care, and with Andrew himself.

In 2009 Offredy et al. carried out a review of case management and long term conditions. While it is recognised that there are many benefits to case management (Table 6.2), their review also highlighted some of the challenges of implementing case management (Table 6.3). These findings are supported by the systematic review undertaken by Sutherland and Hayter in 2009. This review focused on the effectiveness of case management as undertaken by nurses in improving health outcomes in the following LTCs: diabetes, COPD and coronary heart disease.

Core elements	Points to consider	Application to practice
Case finding or screening	Identifying people, through the use of referral criteria, who may benefit from a case management approach. Be aware of hidden populations, e.g., homeless, asylum seekers and travellers. Some examples of referral criteria include: • must be over 18 years of age; • people who frequently use health/social care services; • people who have had two or more accident and emergency and/or hospital admissions in the past 12 months; • people who have one or more LTC; • people who are taking four or more medications.	Andrew has had two unplanned hospital admissions in the last three months. When at home he has a care package for assistance with his personal hygiene and a neighbour cooks meals and helps with housework. Andrew currently takes both a long-acting and a short-acting bronchodilator via a metered dose inhaler and spacer. Due to his recent hospital admissions as a result of a chest infection, he has recently been started on inhaled corticosteroids and is completing a course of antibiotics. His current health status means that he is eligible for a case management approach to his care and management.
Assessment	Assessing a person's health and social care needs using recognised assessments. Using information gathered from the person, their carer and family and other services involved in the person's care. Be aware of obtaining consent to share information and confidentiality. This may include undertaking a physical health assessment, making a diagnosis and non-medical prescribing.	Working with Andrew, David will assess his current health and social care needs, including his concordance and compliance with his medication regime. Given Andrew's current health status this is likely to include a physical health assessment. David will review the current level of support to ensure it is meeting Andrew's health and social care needs. Areas highlighted in David's assessment may include improving his nutritional intake and educating Andrew about the signs that indicate his condition is deteriorating.

continued overleaf...

continued...

Core elements	Points to consider	Application to practice
Care planning	Formulating a personalised care plan to meet the needs identified in the assessment. This care plan may also address anticipated needs. If required, the care plan is agreed with the person's GP and consultant. Coordinates input from other members of the health and social care team may also have some clinical input.	This will depend on the result of Andrew's assessment; it will be David's responsibility to coordinate the input of other agencies. David may refer Andrew on for further nutritional support; David may be required to prescribe nutritional supplements. David is also likely to provide Andrew with information regarding his condition.
Implementation of care plan	Maintaining contact with the person and monitoring input from other health and social care professionals. Provides clinical care if required.	David will become Andrew's single point of contact; he will remain visible to Andrew, ensuring that the care plan is well coordinated. David may also undertake ongoing monitoring of Andrew's physical health status.
Monitoring and reviewing	Monitoring the effectiveness of the care plan and reviewing the level of care if required. Using care pathways and protocols to streamline care.	David will review Andrew's care plan on a regular basis, depending on his current health status. David may use care pathways to support Andrew's care, e.g. acute exacerbation of COPD care pathway.

Table 6.1: Application of the core elements of case management (as described by Hutt et al., 2004) to your clinical practice

This review found, like Offredy et al., that case management was effective in improving a person's level of self-care, increasing their level of psychosocial support and, through effective assessment and monitoring, the progression of their LTC was managed more effectively.

As you can see from Tables 6.2 and 6.3, despite the barriers and challenges to implementing case management, case management provides clear benefits to both those living with an LTC and their carers. Both Offredy et al. (2009) and Sutherland and Hayter (2009) acknowledge that more research into the effectiveness of case management needs to be undertaken, especially in relation to: identifying what specific interventions were the most effective, e.g. non-medical prescribing, finding out if other healthcare professionals could function as community matrons and the effect of case management on long term health and quality of life.

Benefits for those living with an LTC	Benefits for carers and those living with an LTC
Improved physical care, e.g. physical health examinations, assessments and non-medical prescribing, were seen to improve communication and increase trust.	*Education and advice*: both carers and those living with an LTC found the education provided by their case manager/community matron regarding health promotion, disease information and support services increased their ability to self-care, improved their symptom control and minimised ill health.
Care coordination: this was seen to improve the provision of health and social care services, with duplication and gaps in services being minimised.	*Psychosocial support:* case managers and community matrons were seen by both those living with an LTC and their carers as someone that they could depend on.

Table 6.2: The benefits of case management in LTCs (based on the categories of Offredy et al., 2009)

	Barriers	Challenges
Organisation	Poor organisational leadership and a lack of financial support to ensure sufficient resources were available. Insufficient time being allocated to case management.	Lack of resources to enable case managers/community matrons to develop the necessary skills and a lack of practice guidelines for case managers/community matrons.
Communication	Difficulty in accessing services, e.g. therapy services and the amount of paperwork required for some referrals.	Blurring of professional boundaries between case managers, community matrons and other members of the health and social care team could result in reduced or duplicated communication.
Case manager/ community matron	Case managers/community matrons may find it difficult to move from traditional reactive care to a more proactive approach to care; rather than responding to a crisis they prevent a crisis occurring.	Maintaining case loads to a manageable size, increased case loads may mean that the case manager/community matron is not able to participate in activities promoting their personal and professional development.
Patient	The complexity of the person's health and social care needs.	Difficulty in maintaining a person's healthy lifestyles.

Table 6.3: Some of the barriers and challenges to implementing case management (based on the categories of Offredy et al., 2009)

Reflecting back on your recent clinical experience identify a person, living with an LTC, who had complex care needs and compile a map or diagram of the services involved in their care and management.

Using the information provided in Table 6.1 apply the core elements to your chosen person and review how case management could have improved their care and management.

As the answers will be based on your own observations there is no outline answer at the end of this chapter.

As discussed above, Activity 6.2 will have demonstrated to you how, through ensuring an appropriate and responsive plan of care is in place, case management can be used to improve the care and management of people living with an LTC. In your current role you may not be actively involved in case management; however, using the information in Table 6.1 in your nursing practice will support you in your delivery of effective care to people living with an LTC.

Managing complex care

For some people living with an LTC it is inevitable that as their condition deteriorates their health and social care needs will become increasingly more complex. As mentioned in Chapter 1 of this book (page 9) the main policy documents concerning LTCs emphasise the important role primary care services have in managing the care of people living with an LTC, including those with complex needs. This includes managing acute exacerbations. For those involved in this aspect of the care and management of this group of people, like case managers, there are some useful resources available to support them in their delivery of person-centred care. One such resource is integrated care pathways (ICPs). ICPs are also known as care pathways and maps of care, but for consistency the term integrated care pathway (ICP) will be used in this chapter.

Integrated care pathways and LTCs

An integrated care pathway is a multidisciplinary outline of anticipated care for patients with a similar diagnosis or set of symptoms. The ICP document specifies the interventions required for the patient to progress along the pathway and places them against a timeframe measured in terms of hours, days, weeks or milestones.

(Middleton et al., 2001, page 2)

ICPs are focused on the needs of the person in relation to where they are on their journey through healthcare services. The aim of ICPs is to improve both the coordination and consistency of care a person receives. They allow you to *deliver the right care to the right person in the right place and at the right time*. ICPs tend to have some common themes. They are multidisciplinary, meaning that they are written and used by all members of the health and social care team. This single point of communication has the potential to lead to improved communication and coordination of care. They are designed for a specific group of people, e.g. those in the last few days or hours of their life. For this specific group of people the Liverpool Care Pathway for the Dying Patient is used. As a student nurse you may have used this care pathway to support the care you deliver to people in the last few days or hours of their life. This care pathway can be used in a variety of setting, e.g. nursing home or secondary care setting. Using this pathway will ensure that you deliver the best quality care to those who are dying, regardless of the clinical setting. Finally, and most importantly, ICPs include the care to be delivered, what the aim of that care is and the timeframe within which it is to be met (Middleton et al., 2001).

It should be noted, however, that while ICPs form the template of the care to be delivered, the people receiving the care are individuals and will not all respond in the same way and follow the same pathway of care. It is necessary therefore that these individualities are accommodated within the ICP. These individualities are known as 'variances'. Variances allow for healthcare professionals to use their professional judgement in relation to the care being delivered. Recognising and managing variances requires you, as a student nurse, to be able to problem solve. Using the nursing process as discussed in Chapter 5 will support you in your ability to do this. When a variance is noted, the following should be recorded on the care pathway: what variance occurred and why, the action taken (personalised care plan) and the outcome of the action. The aim of the action taken in relation to a variance is to return the person to the ICP as soon as possible (Middleton et al., 2001). Table 6.4 outlines how the nursing process can be applied to ICPs and managing variances in a person's care.

The nursing process	Integrated care pathway	Application to practice
Assess	You are using the Liverpool Care Pathway for the Dying Patient to guide the care you deliver to a person in the last few days of their life. Currently you are undertaking an initial assessment regarding their skin integrity.	You use a recognised risk assessment tool, e.g. the Waterlow pressure ulcer risk assessment tool, to assess the person's skin.
Systematic nursing diagnosis	This assessment gives you a risk score of 22, indicating that the person has a very high risk of developing a pressure ulcer.	
Plan	You record the result of your assessment on the initial assessment sheet to ensure that all members of the healthcare team are aware of the results of your assessment. You use these results to plan your care and to set appropriate goals.	The results of your assessment indicate that the following preventative pressure reducing equipment is needed: • when in bed an appropriate alternating pressure mattress is used. *— continued overleaf...*

continued...

The nursing process	Integrated care pathway	Application to practice
Implement	In addition to using appropriate pressure reducing equipment, working with the person you implement a care plan and set goals that address the following aspects of nursing care: • general nursing care – regular positional changes; • pain – any pain is being assessed and well controlled; • nutrition – a high protein nutritious diet is available; • person handling – the correct moving and lifting techniques are used; • skin care – good personal hygiene, ensuring that the skin in kept clean and dry. This is recorded on the initial assessment sheet. As per instructions on the Liverpool Care Pathway for the Dying Patient, it is agreed that this care will be rechecked every four hours.	
Recheck	You record, on the ongoing assessment of the plan of care, the person's skin integrity, recording their Waterlow score and identifying if their skin integrity is maintained. You record this change on both the ongoing assessment of the plan of care and the variance analysis sheet.	During one of your checks you notice a change in skin integrity. There is a change in skin colour on the right heel: the skin is intact; however, non-blanching erythema is present. As a grade one pressure ulcer is classed as a wound you implement a care plan to address this. This includes: • regular positional changes; • ensuring that there is no pressure on the right heel; • applying a film or thin hydrocolloid dressing for protection.
Evaluate	Using the care pathway, and identified care plan to address the grade one pressure ulcer, ensures that evaluation takes place every four hours. This evaluation consists of: • ongoing pressure ulcer risk assessment; • ongoing review of the care plan.	

Table 6.4: Application of the nursing process and an integrated care pathway to your clinical practice

As you can see from Table 6.4, by providing you with a clear framework within which to work, both the nursing process and ICPs are useful resources to use to support your delivery of person-centred care.

Activity 6.3   *Evidence-based practice and research*

During your next practice learning experience, with the support of your mentor, find the ICPs that are used to support care; these could be local or national. Review a selection of these integrated care pathways and consider the following questions.

- Is there a clear evidence base presented for the ICP?
- Is there a regular review date?
- Is the ICP linked to other policy within the trust?
- Is there clear guidance on how to complete the ICP?
- Is the ICP easy to navigate: do you know where to document your initial assessment, ongoing care and variances?

If your answer is no to any of the above questions, discuss this with your mentor and identify how you could improve the ICP.

As the answers will be based on your own observations there is no outline answer at the end of this chapter.

ICPs not only support the delivery of responsive person-centred care, they also can be used to support the delivery of cost-effective care. Map of Medicine is an online resource that aims to support the delivery of high quality healthcare, in line with the aims of the Department of Health's 2010 publication (DH, 2010b), *The NHS Quality, Innovation, Productivity and Prevention Challenge: An Introduction for Clinicians.*

Their online resources include information on the following:

- how the maps of care have been shown to improve patient outcome, reduce delivery costs and support efficient service delivery;
- how the maps of care have been used to support the commissioning of services;
- how healthcare professionals and communities have been using maps of care to develop the services they provide;
- an extensive range of care maps accessible to all members of the healthcare team.

Each map is supported by an appropriate evidence base including research and clinical guidelines from the National Institute for Health and Clinical Excellence (NICE), the Scottish Intercollegiate Guidelines Network (SIGN) and others. This ensures that the information provided is based on best available evidence and is suitable for use throughout the UK. While the maps are not as detailed as an ICP they do provide information regarding treatment options and where care should be delivered, e.g. in primary or secondary care. As well as providing the above information for healthcare professionals, Map of Medicine also provides health guides. These are evidence-based, easy-to-use guides that people receiving care for a specific LTC, or their family/carer, can access.

Case study: Frazer

Frazer is now 50 and has been living with his Type 1 diabetes since he was 8. He lives with his long term partner Claire and their daughter Fiona, who is now 14. He was diagnosed with diabetic polyneuropathy

continued overleaf...

• continued... •

10 years ago. Despite improving his level of foot care and maintaining reasonable blood glucose control, between 6 and 9 mmol/l before meals, Frazer has had ongoing problems with foot ulceration, and over the past few days he has been feeling unwell and has had a slight temperature. He has also found it harder to maintain his blood glucose levels and these have been slightly raised at between 9 and 11 mmol/l before meals.

Today while inspecting his feet he has noticed that the area round the ulcer on his right foot is red and swollen. Today he is unable to put his shoes on due to the swelling. He phones his GP and makes an appointment to see him today.

Frazer's GP accesses Map of Medicine to support his decision-making process: he accesses the diabetes foot care map and follows the map for infection. On assessment it is evident to his GP that Frazer's ulcer has become infected, and to ensure appropriate treatment and management Frazer's GP refers him for an expert assessment within one working day.

The following day Frazer attends his local diabetic foot clinic, where he is assessed by members of the team. The team at the diabetic foot clinic also access Map of Medicine to ensure appropriate treatment. It is evident from their assessment and investigations that the infection is severe (graded three using PEDIS) and will need to be treated with a broad spectrum intravenous antibiotic. As a result of this Frazer is admitted to hospital for intravenous antibiotic therapy, daily wound care and review.

Frazer remained on intravenous antibiotics for 48 hours; he spent three days in hospital. On discharge he was to continue taking oral antibiotics for three weeks and was referred to the diabetic foot clinic for ongoing review, with an emphasis being placed on self-management and regular chiropody appointments.

Case management improves the care and management of people living with an LTC and through preventative interventions can reduce admission to secondary care. But managing an acute exacerbation of their condition in primary care may not always be possible for people living with an LTC (as Frazer's situation suggests). For people living with an LTC, and their carers, admission to secondary care can be a time of stress and anxiety. Hospital admission can place a person at risk of hospital-acquired infection; it can often result in a reduction in a person's functional ability, especially in the elderly and those with a cognitive impairment, and can increase a person's social isolation.

Research summary: Dementia and secondary care

For people with dementia, removal from their familiar surroundings where they may just be able to 'cope', to an unfamiliar setting where it is busy and there are lots of new faces, can be bewildering. It is known that up to 97% of nurses in a secondary (or tertiary) care setting are responsible for caring for people with dementia (Alzheimer's Society, 2009). In a busy ward environment people with dementia can be seen as being 'challenging' to nurses: they require more time to be spent with them, they may display unpredictable behaviour, they may wander, and communication with them can be difficult. From the perspective of the carer, findings from the Alzheimer's Society's report (2009) noted that up to 47% of carers said that admission to secondary care had a negative effect on the

continued opposite...

continued...

physical health of the individual with dementia and 54% of carers said that an admission to secondary care had a negative effect on the symptoms of dementia, for example increased confusion and changes in behaviour. It is important, therefore, for both nurses and those with dementia, that strategies are in place to support nurses to maximise care and to ensure that for those living with dementia any deterioration in their condition is minimised. Strategies that have been identified include the following (Heath, 2010).

*   Improving orientation to the environment – this requires a committed approach from hospital management. Improving lighting, reducing noise and providing signposting, especially to toilets, can improve a person's orientation. Personalising a person's bed space and locker will enable them to identify it easily and will provide reassurance.
*   Using a 'This is Me' guide and/or memory books (see Chapter 4) – these are simple and practical tools that provide an overview of the person with dementia. 'This is Me' addresses areas such as the person's ability to manage their activities of daily living, their likes and dislikes and what worries them. For information on memory books see the section on self-management for people living with dementia in Chapter 4 of this book.
*   Learning from carers – as previously mentioned in this book, carers play an important role in supporting people living with an LTC, and it is important to use their knowledge of the person to inform the care you are providing. Carers may also be willing to participate in a person's care, for example, helping them to eat at meal times, though you will need to take into consideration the privacy of other patients in the ward should this happen.
*   Improving communication – finding suitable ways of communication with people who have dementia will improve the quality of care given. Observing the person and talking to their carer will enable the most appropriate method to be found, for example, using pictures, and observing facial expressions and body postures. By speaking clearly, keeping language simple, using the person's name consistently and demonstrating warmth, communication can be improved and levels of understanding increased.

The strategies identified above, such as working with carers, improving communication, learning about the person and effective pain assessment and management (see Chapter 5, page 96) have the potential to minimise the risk of challenging behaviours occurring. However, it is acknowledged that episodes of challenging behaviour may still occur, and using the ABC approach to assess challenging behaviour can support effective management.

*   A – Antecedents/triggers, what was happening before the challenging behaviour occurred? Who was present and where did it happen?
*   B – Behaviour, what challenging behaviour occurred? Has this happened before or is this behaviour new?
*   C – Consequences, what happened as a result of this behaviour?

Using the strategies outlined above will improve the care delivered to those with dementia, and their carers, whilew in secondary care. By working to minimise any deterioration in

continued overleaf...

continued...

a person's level of cognitive ability and supporting and working with carers, appropriate and timely discharge can be achieved.

The following article and website provide more information:

Heath, H. (2010) Improving the quality of care for people with dementia in general hospitals. *Quality of Care Supplement*.1–16.

www.alzheimers.org.uk/countingthecost. This site contains information about the Alzheimer's Society's campaign to improve the quality of care for those with dementia who are admitted to secondary care.

It is important, when caring for those living with an LTC in a secondary care setting, to ensure that effective discharge planning is in place. Effective discharge has the potential to minimise a person's length of stay in secondary care, reducing the risk of complications mentioned above arising.

Discharge planning in LTCs

The important role discharge planning plays has been recognised by the NHS Institute for Innovation and Improvement (2010) in their *High Impact Actions for Nursing and Midwifery: The Essential Collection*. The High Impact Actions represent the areas of care where poor patient experience is evident, and they include:

- your skin matters;
- staying safe – preventing falls;
- keeping nourished – getting better;
- promoting normal birth;
- important choices – where to die when the time comes;
- fit and well to care;
- ready to go – no delays;
- protection from infection.

Further information on the High Impact Actions is available from the NHS Institute for Innovation and Improvement website listed at the end of this chapter.

Discharge planning is not an isolated event: it should be a process that is started when a person is admitted to secondary care. Starting discharge planning early allows both the person being discharged and their carer to be involved in the process as much as possible. There is not scope in this chapter to address all aspects of discharge planning, therefore the remainder of this section will focus on the role of ensuring effective medication management in discharge planning and the importance of involving carers in the discharge process. These two areas have been chosen as it is recognised that successful medicines management is an important aspect of care and management of LTCs (see Chapter 5) and that informal carers play a pivotal role in supporting people living with an LTC (see Chapters 1, 2 and 3). However, to increase your knowledge and understanding of the discharge process take the time to undertake Activity 6.4. This activity will allow you to examine a local discharge policy/protocol and explore some of the reasons why discharge planning is successful or not.

Activity 6.4   *Evidence-based practice and research*

During your next practice learning experience locate your local discharge policy/ protocol and associated documentation, for example discharge check list, and familiarise yourself with it. Then answer the following questions.

1. Is the discharge policy/protocol followed?

If you answer yes to this questions then go to question 2; if you answered no then go to question 3.
2. Why is this – are there specific strategies/attitudes in place to ensure it is followed?
3. Why is this – what prevents the discharge policy/protocol being followed?

If you answered question 2 then go to question 4, if you answered question 3 then go to question 5.
4. How could this area of good practice be shared with other clinical areas?
5. What could be done to improve the discharge planning process in this area?

As the answers will be based on your own observations there is no outline answer at the end of this chapter.

Self-administration of medicines to aid the discharge planning process

When a person living with an LTC is admitted to secondary care it is important, where possible, that they maintain their self-management role in relation to their medication. This approach promotes their independence and contributes to their discharge planning. In order to support people to do this each NHS Trust will have their own locally agreed policy relating to self-administration of medicines. However, there will be some common criteria contained in these (NPC, 2007c):

- that the person's own medication should be used;
- that an accurate assessment of the person's ability to self-administer is undertaken;
- that lockable bedside storage for the person's medication should be available.

Within a trust policy there may be varying levels of self-administration, for example:

- level three – here the person self-administers their medication and is given responsibility for the key to the medicine locker during their stay in hospital;
- level two – the person administers their medication with supervision and the key for the medicine locker in held by the nursing staff;
- level one – the person's medication is administered by the nursing staff with a full explanation; this is similar to the traditional method of administration.

Activity 6.5   *Critical thinking*

Case scenario: Angela

Angela is now 39 years old and has been living with relapsing remitting multiple sclerosis (RRMS) since she was 28. During this current relapse Angela has been experiencing visual impairment and double vision with some loss of balance. She has been admitted to secondary care for intravenous corticosteroids. Her current medication consists of:

- baclofen: 20 mg three times a day;
- paracetamol: two tablets up to four times a day for pain relief;
- movicol: one sachet daily.

At home Angela is able to take her medication independently; however, due to her double vision and visual impairment her medication is being dispensed by the ward staff. Angela is not experiencing any difficulty with her manual dexterity, though she does have some difficulty in reading at the moment and with her perception of distance. Angela is keen to begin to take responsibility for her medication again and asks you if it is possible for her to self-administer her own medication in preparation for her discharge home.

To help you undertake this activity find your local trust policy relating to self-administration of medication, and use this policy to do the following:

- assess Angela's ability to administer her own medication;
- plan when you would next review Angela regarding her self-administration of medication;
- once this has been done provide Angela with the relevant information about self-administration of medication.

You may also wish to consider the following.

- Who would usually carry out this assessment and how often is it reviewed?
- Are carers involved in this assessment?

As the answers will be based on your own observations there is no outline answer at the end of this chapter.

As you will have seen from Activity 6.5, in order for self-administration to be successful the person involved needs to be assessed and reviewed appropriately and provided with the relevant information. Self-administration of medication in the care and management of LTCs while a person is receiving hospital care maintains their level of independence, promotes self-management and contributes to their discharge planning. Working with people who are self-administering their medication will assist you to improve your knowledge of medication management, as you will be required to provide a clear explanation of when to take their medication, what their medication does and what the side-effects are.

Involving carers in the discharge process

By involving carers in the discharge planning process you are recognising the important role they play in supporting the person living with an LTC. They may have been a carer for many years and have built up an excellent knowledge and understanding of the needs of the person they are caring for. For others they may be new to caring and have concerns about how they are going to manage in this new role when the person is discharged. Not all people choose to be carers; many find themselves taking on this role over a period of months or years. To ensure a smooth discharge it is important therefore to find out how willing and able a person is to undertake care activities, for example how is their own health, and do they require information or support about their role as a carer. As mentioned in Chapter 2 carers, under The Carers (Recognition and Services) Act 1995, The Carers and Disabled Children Act 2000 and The Carers (Equal Opportunities) Act 2004, have the right to an assessment of their needs. Offering carers this assessment before the person they care for is discharged will ensure that appropriate support is in place and that any concerns are highlighted.

Communication with carers is key in promoting a discharge planning process that includes the carer; a person's carer should be identified on admission with the carer's details and current caring input being included in the admission documentation. Carers are, on admission, able to provide useful and necessary information on a person's condition should they not be able to communicate themselves, for example due to a neurological LTC or confusion. This information can then be used to inform care planning and discharge planning (Princess Royal Trust for Carers, 2010). Communicating with and involving carers in the discharge planning process can provide them with realistic expectations about what to expect on discharge, for example regarding disease progression, preparing them for their role and ensuring adequate support is in place. It is also important to provide ongoing support following discharge to support the carer in their role. Useful information and advice regarding information and support is available in Chapter 2 of this book in the section covering the therapeutic relationship and carers.

Conclusion

Having read this chapter, worked through the activities and accessed the further reading you will have developed your knowledge and skills in relation to how complex care, in LTCs, is managed. How you use this new knowledge will depend on where you work and your roles and responsibilities. However, as a nurse you can contribute to the complex care of people living with an LTC. By having an awareness and understanding of the role and responsibilities of the case manager you can liaise effectively with members of the multidisciplinary team to provide an appropriate level of care. By accessing and using ICPs you can ensure that those living with LTCs receive evidence-based care. Recognising the importance of the discharge planning process will enable you to work with those living with an LTC and their carers to address relevant concerns and issues.

Chapter summary

This chapter has provided you with an overview of complex care in LTCs and how it is managed. It has outlined the important role case management plays in promoting proactive care and in increasing satisfaction in those living with an LTC. It has related the roles and responsibilities of the case manager to one of the case scenarios you

continued overleaf...

• • *continued...* •

have been following in this book, allowing you to see the integration of theory to your clinical practice. ICPs have been explored in relation to the care and management of those with LTCs; using ICPs ensures that an appropriate plan of care is provided. The importance of discharge planning has been highlighted with the emphasis being placed on promoting self-administration of medicines for those living with an LTC and recognising carers in the discharge planning process. Finally some specific strategies for supporting discharge in those with a cognitive impairment have been discussed.

Further reading

Borthwick, R, Newbronner, L and Stuttard, L (2009) 'Out of Hospital': a scoping study of services for carers of people being discharged from hospital. *Health and Social Care in the Community*, 17 (4): 335–49.
This article summarises a scoping study aimed at identifying the service provision for carers during the discharge process and at the point of discharge.

Department of Health (2010) *Ready to Go? Planning the Discharge and Transfer of Patients from Hospital and Intermediate Care*. Leeds: Department of Health.
This guide explains the ten key steps to achieving a safe and timely discharge, and is aimed at both health and social care professionals.

Kempshall, N (2010) The care of patients with complex long-term conditions. *British Journal of Community Nursing*, 15 (4): 18 –87.
This article provides an overview of case management in LTCs and relates it to a case study.

Useful websites

www.mapofmedicine.com
This website provides information on care pathways and outlines the care pathways for a range of LTCs, addressing all aspects of care from diagnosis, through to managing acute exacerbations and end-of-life care.

http://healthguides.mapofmedicine.com/choices/map/index.html
This website is linked to **www.mapofmedicine.com** and contains evidence-based, easy-to-use guides that people living with an LTC, their carer or family can access.

www.institute.nhs.uk/building_capability/general/aims.html
The home page for High Impact Actions: The Essential Collection. It contains useful information and examples of case studies.

Chapter 7
Palliative care in long term conditions

NMC Standards for Pre-registration Nursing Education

This chapter will address the following competencies:

Domain 1: Professional values

1.1 Adult nurses must understand and apply current legislation to all service users, paying special attention to the protection of vulnerable people, including those with complex needs arising from ageing, cognitive impairment, long term conditions and those approaching the end-of-life.

5. All nurses must fully understand the nurse's various roles, responsibilities and functions, and adapt their practice to meet the changing needs of people, groups, communities and populations.

Domain 3: Nursing practice and decision-making

4. All nurses must ascertain and respond to the physical, social and psychological needs of people, groups and communities. They must then plan, deliver and evaluate safe, competent, person-centred care in partnerships with them, paying special attention to changing health needs during different life stages, including progressive illness and death, loss and bereavement.

4.2 Adult nurses must recognise and respond to the changing needs of adults, families and carers during terminal illness. They must be aware of how treatment goals and service users' choices may change at different stages of progressive illness, loss and bereavement.

NMC Essential Skills Clusters

This chapter will address the following ESCs:

Cluster: Care, compassion and communication

6. People can trust the newly registered graduate nurse to engage therapeutically and actively listen to their needs and concerns, responding using skills that are helpful, providing information that is clear, accurate, meaningful and free from jargon.

By entry to the register

13. Uses appropriate and relevant communication skills to deal with difficult and challenging circumstances, for example, responding to emergencies, unexpected occurrences, saying 'no', dealing with complaints, resolving disputes, de-escalating aggression, conveying 'unwelcome news'.

continued overleaf...

• • *continued...* •

Cluster: Organisational aspects of care

9. People can trust the newly registered graduate nurse to treat them as partners and work with them to make a holistic and systematic assessment of their needs; to develop a personalised plan that is based on mutual understanding and respect for their individual situation promoting health and wellbeing, minimising risk of harm and promoting their safety at all times.

By entry to the register

16. Promotes health and wellbeing, self-care and independence by teaching and empowering people and carers to make choices in coping with the effects of treatment and the ongoing nature and likely consequences of a condition including death and dying.

Chapter aims

After reading this chapter you will be able to:

- discuss and apply the principles of breaking bad news to the care and management of people living with an LTC;
- explain what palliative care is and its role in the management of LTCs;
- explain the end-of-life care strategy and its relevance to people living with an LTC;
- recognise the importance of advance care planning in the management of LTCs.

Introduction

You matter to us because you are you, and you matter to the last moment of your life. We will do all we can not only to help you die peacefully, but also to live until you die.

(Dame Cicely Saunders (1994))

As mentioned in Chapter 1, the incidence of LTCs is rising; there are many LTCs where the trajectory of the condition is such that there will come a time when all active treatment options have been tried. It is at this point in a person's journey when their treatment and care moves from active to palliative. For some this may not be for many years as appropriate health promotion, effective self-care and symptom management slow down the progression of their LTC and its impact on them and their life. For others, such as those diagnosed with a rapidly progressing neurological disorder or a specific cancer, where any treatment will be non-curative, palliative care may be a more immediate part of their care and management. Whether the transition from active to palliative treatment comes late or early in a person's journey, it is important that they are provided with the knowledge to enable them to make informed decisions about their care and that they are able to communicate their fears and desires to those caring for them.

Talking about death and dying is not something we are comfortable about as it reminds us of our own mortality; however, effectively supporting people receiving palliative care requires you to become involved and empathise with the person and their situation. Utilising the knowledge and skills developed in Chapter 2 will enable you to recognise your own fears as well as those of the people in your care, allowing you to effectively support both individuals living with an LTC and those who care for them.

As the above quote emphasises, palliative care is about focusing on the person and enabling them to carry on 'living' while receiving palliative care. The move from active to palliative treatment is not seen as the end of the journey but rather as a new approach to care. To support you in caring for people during the transition from active to palliative treatment, and the areas to be considered, this chapter will assist you in your development of the knowledge and skills required to enable those in the end stages of their life to live their life and die in the place of their choice and in a manner appropriate for them. In order to do this, the chapter will help you develop your knowledge, skills and attributes in relation to breaking bad news, palliative care and planning for end-of-life care including advance care planning.

Policy review

Traditionally palliative care has been part of the care and management of people living with cancer; however, changes in demographics and the increase in LTCs (see Chapter 1) have meant that palliative care is now seen as part of the care and management of any person living with a life-threatening condition. There is also available evidence that suggests that not all people living with an LTC receive appropriate palliative care, with areas such as deteriorating health, social isolation, carer burden and lack of access to services being highlighted as areas of concern (Fitzsimons et al., 2007). Given this it is essential therefore that planning for, and providing palliative care for, people living with an LTC, and their carer and family, is a key component of the care and management of LTCs. This may mean that a person in the end stages of living with dementia is supported at home by their Admiral nurse, GP, district nurse team and social care professionals with specialist palliative care support from the local hospice. A person living with lung cancer may be supported at home by their Macmillan nurse, district nursing team and GP with access to hospice day services and in-patient services should the person request them. To reflect this palliative care has been included in the *National Service Framework (NSF) for Long Term Conditions* (Department of Health (DH), 2005a) quality requirement 9: palliative care; the aim of this being to ensure that people living with an LTC receive holistic end-of-life care that addresses their physical, social, psychological and spiritual needs. In Scotland, *Long Term Conditions Collaborative: High Impact Changes* (NHS Scotland, 2009) addresses aspects of palliative care in High Impact Changes 2 and 5. High Impact Change 2 includes planning for the future, and addresses such issues as advance care planning for end of life. High Impact Change 5 states that as much care as possible, including end-of-life care, should be delivered close to or in the person's home. While policy documents, focusing on LTCs, in Northern Ireland (Long Term Conditions Alliance Northern Ireland, 2008) and Wales (Department of Health and Social Services, 2007) do not specifically mention the role of palliative care, their underlying ethos of providing the right care at the right time and in the right place implicitly includes palliative care as part of the care and management of LTCs. As well as supporting the integration of palliative care as part of the care and management of people living with an LTC, all countries in the UK have published strategies outlining the role of palliative care in healthcare:

- Wales: *A Strategic Direction for Palliative Care Services in Wales* (Welsh Assembly Government (WAG), 2003); this strategy is supported by the following website: http://wales.pallcare.info/index.php;
- Scotland: *Living and Dying Well: a national action plan for palliative and end of life care in Scotland* (The Scottish Government (TSG), 2008);
- England: *End of Life Care Strategy: Promoting high quality care for all adults at the end of life* (DH, 2008e), this strategy is supported by the following website: **www.endoflifecareforadults.nhs.uk/**;
- Northern Ireland: *Palliative and End of Life Care Strategy for Northern Ireland: Consultation Document* (Department of Health, Social Services and Public Safety (DHSSPS), 2009).

The above strategies state that people requiring palliative care should receive appropriate and timely treatment that is holistic and delivered in a place of their choice.

Breaking bad news in long term conditions

Chapter 1 introduced you to the concept of physical and psychological 'noise' in your communication with people living with an LTC. The impact of 'noise' was discussed in relation to the delivery of a diagnosis of an LTC and its perception as being 'bad news'. In Chapter 1 bad news was described as any news that implies the loss of something, e.g. physical ability, that an individual values, or is life changing affecting an individual's perception of themselves. For many people living with an LTC the move from active to palliative treatment will be seen as further bad news, and this is compounded by the fact that they are now faced with the realisation that they are entering the final stages of their journey. Breaking bad news is a complex but necessary part of the care and management of people living with an LTC. As well as breaking the bad news the person has to prepare themselves for the emotional reaction of the person and their family. They will have to be prepared to answer questions, such as, 'how long do I have?', 'is there anything else that can be done?', provide information regarding future care and management and ensure that they have been understood by the person receiving the bad news. Although breaking bad news can be difficult and unpleasant for both the healthcare professional and the person receiving the news, it is important. It helps to maintain trust in the therapeutic relationship, reduces uncertainty ('at least I know what I am dealing with'), prevents the build-up of inappropriate hope ('is there something I should be doing?'), allows the person and their family time to adjust and allows for open communication between the healthcare professionals, the person and their family (Kaye, 1996).

Activity 7.1   *Reflection*

Whether it is breaking bad news or answering awkward questions, many healthcare professionals find this difficult to do. Either on your own or with a group of your peers, reflect back on your clinical experience and identify a situation where you have been

continued opposite...

continued... •
asked an awkward question that you did not feel comfortable answering. Now answer the
following questions.

- What was it about the situation that made it awkward?
- How did you respond to the person's question?
- Would you do it differently now?

As the answers will be based on your own observations there is no outline answer at the end of this chapter.

Activity 7.1 will have demonstrated to you that there are many reasons why healthcare
professionals feel uncomfortable when breaking bad news or answering awkward questions.
They are reminded of their own mortality, they are worried about saying the wrong thing or
they are unprepared for the reaction of the person. Some questions (Kaye, 1996) that may be
useful for you to use in a similar situation to the one reflected on in Activity 7.1 are as follows.

- 'What makes you ask me this question?'
- 'What do you already know about your condition?'
- 'Would it help you to know more about your condition?'
- 'Would you like to have a member of your family with you when you find out more about
  your condition?'

This approach will enable you to explore the person's concerns without having to give information
that you may not feel capable or competent to deliver. Given the complexities of breaking bad
news, some approaches have been developed to support and guide the process (Kaye,1996; Baile
et al., 2000).

Approaches to use when breaking bad news in LTCs

Bad news should be delivered in a sensitive manner, allowing the person to feel that they have
been listened to and understood. The person, and their carer and family, should leave knowing
what the plan for their future care and treatment is. To support healthcare professionals in
breaking bad news, specific approaches have been developed. Perhaps the best known method
is Kaye's 10 steps to breaking bad news (1996); another method is Baile et al.'s SPIKES 6 step
protocol (2000), which is similar to Kaye's 10 step approach. Table 7.1 outlines both Kaye's 10
steps to breaking bad news (1996) and Baile et al.'s SPIKES 6 step protocol (2000) and applies
them to your practice.

Kaye's 10 steps to breaking bad news (Kaye, 1996)	SPIKES 6 step protocol (Baile et al., 2000)	Areas to consider
1. Preparation	Setting	Know all the facts before the consultation; ensure privacy and comfort. Check that all the appropriate people are there; 'Is there anyone with you today that you would like to be part

continued overleaf...

continued...

Kaye's 10 steps to breaking bad news (Kaye, 1996)	SPIKES 6 step protocol (Baile et al., 2000)	Areas to consider
		of this meeting?' Remember in some cultures it would be expected that the head of the family be present.
2. What does the person know?	Perception	Ask for a narrative of events from the person to determine their perception of the illness: 'could you tell me...' or 'how did it all start?' Ask the person what they understand is happening: 'do you know why we are meeting today?'
3. What information is wanted?	Invitation	Obtain permission for the person for more information: 'would you like me to explain a bit more?'. Remember that for the person it can be frightening asking for more information – how much do they want to know?
4. Give a warning shot	Knowledge	Warn first about sharing bad news: 'I'm afraid this is rather serious' or 'the news is not what we had hoped for'. Denial is a natural coping mechanism: allow the person to control how much information is given. Narrow the information gap by providing information in simple language; check understanding before continuing. Avoid being blunt, giving incomplete information or false hope. The detail may not be remembered but how you gave the information will be.
5. Allow denial		
6. Explain (if asked)		
7. Listen to concerns	Emotion	Allow for expression of feelings: 'what are your main concerns at the moment?' Respond with empathy, address the person's concerns and emotions: 'this must be difficult for you'; explore and validate the person's feelings: 'it is only natural that you feel this way'. For the person, this is the most important part in relation to their satisfaction with the meeting.
8. Encourage expression of feelings		

continued opposite...

continued...

| 9. Summary and plan | Summary | Review the information discussed and provide a summary, answer questions, discuss options and plans for future care. Offer availability: some details may not be remembered, further support will be needed and they may need time to talk to family. |
| 10. Offer availability | | |

Table 7.1: Areas to consider when using Kaye's (1996) 10 steps to breaking bad news or Baile et al.'s SPIKES (2000) 6 step protocol

Activity 7.2   *Reflection*

Reflecting back on your recent clinical experience where you have witnessed 'bad news' being broken, were either Kaye's 10 steps to breaking bad news (Kaye 1996) or Baile et al.'s SPIKES 6 step protocol (Baile, 2000) used? If they were used how effective were they? If they were not used, then how would using this protocol have improved the situation?

In the further reading section at the end of this chapter there is an article that supports the use of the SPIKES 6 step protocol when breaking bad news to people with a learning disability.

As the answers will be based on your own observations there is no outline answer at the end of this chapter.

Using the approaches outlined in Table 7.1 should help you to improve the process of breaking bad news, both for the person delivering the bad news and for the person receiving the bad news. When undertaking Activity 7.2 you may have reflected on how the person receiving the bad news reacted to the news. However sensitively bad news is broken the reaction of the person, and their family, to the news can be unpredictable. Knowing the person and how they have reacted to previous bad news will help you to support them during this stage.

Reactions to bad news

From your previous clinical, and life, experiences you will be aware that people react to hearing bad news in a variety of ways. Their initial reactions may include denial ('I don't believe this'), numbness ('this can't be happening'), anger ('I knew there was something wrong, if only the tests had been carried out sooner') and grief. A person's reactions depend on the size of the loss and their usual coping mechanisms. How well they have coped with previous 'bad news' and changes in the status of their LTC will be an indicator as to how well they will cope with the news that their treatment is changing from active to palliative. Many people put on a 'brave face' and, at the time of hearing the news, are able to conduct a rational dialogue, asking for further information and rechecking what has already been said. This is their way of confirming the reality of their situation as psychologically they struggle to come to terms with the news. However, as noted in Table 7.1 it is likely that they will not remember the details of the consultation and the information provided, therefore it is important to review their understanding at a later date. Early reactions to the news such as anger, guilt and sadness may also be present; anger may be expressed towards family and members of the healthcare team (Radziewicz and Baile, 2001). You should remember that the person is not angry with you but at the news that has been delivered. Once the initial reaction to the news has passed, some later reactions and coping mechanisms that people display include:

- fighting spirit – 'I will not let this beat me';
- stoical acceptance – 'this is how it is and I will just have to get on with it';
- denial – 'there is nothing wrong with me';
- resigned helplessness – 'what is the point in doing anything, the damage is already done'.

Research summary: 'Fighting spirit' and 'denial'

Research has been undertaken in relation to 'fighting spirit' and 'denial' in people with a diagnosis of cancer. The findings of this research suggest that those who cope with either a fighting spirit or denial might survive longer (Greer, 1999), though the evidence has been challenged (Watson et al., 1999). Greer demonstrated a statistically significant correlation between fighting spirit and cancer survival: Watson et al. found no such correlation but did note that depression and hopelessness had a modest, negative, impact on disease outcome. Greer argued that this supported her results as hopelessness is the polar opposite of fighting spirit (Greer et al., 2000). O'Baugh et al. (2003) noted that being 'positive' for patients meant maintaining some sort of normality, and not letting the cancer have a negative impact on daily life. However, for nurses it meant having a 'fighting spirit' and wanting to get through the treatment. This mismatch has the potential to have a negative impact on the therapeutic relationship and any communication between the nurse and patient. For example, being positive, from the patient's perspective, may mean they are perceived as being 'awkward', wanting treatment to be scheduled round their lives and not vice versa. Nurses therefore need to know what their patients mean by 'being positive' in relation to themselves and their illness, and incorporate this into their care planning and management.

As you can see from the box above extensive research has been done into the many aspects of people's responses to bad news and the realisation that their care is moving from active to palliative. Perhaps the most definitive work in this area is that of Elisabeth Kübler-Ross who in 1969 completed a study that focused on people's reactions to their own dying and death. During this study she interviewed over 200 people about their thoughts and feelings in relation to their dying and death. The result of this work was the five stages of dying: denial, anger, bargaining, depression and acceptance (Kübler-Ross, 2009). It should be noted that Kübler-Ross emphasised that these were the stages people may go through and that they may not progress through them in a linear manner.

The stages have evolved since their introduction, and they have been very misunderstood over the past three decades. They were never meant to help tuck messy emotions into neat packages. They are responses to loss that many people have, but there is not a typical response to loss, as there is no typical loss. Our grief is as individual as our lives. Not everyone goes through all of them or in a prescribed order.

Kübler-Ross (2005, page 7)

Over time the stages of dying have been applied to those who are grieving; however, their relevance to grieving has been questioned (Friedman and James, 2008). To support you in your care of the bereaved there are many available bereavement theories. See also the further reading list at the end of this chapter.

At whatever point in the course of a person's illness bad news is broken, what is important is that their ongoing palliative care needs are met. However, for the progression of some LTCs (e.g. COPD, heart failure), it can be difficult to predict and many people will have lived through many exacerbations of their condition. For example, it is estimated that up to 50% of people with heart failure will die suddenly (Wilmot, 2002). It is essential therefore to ensure that the relevant care and management is in place early for these people, allowing for maximum symptom relief and quality of life.

Palliative care

Palliative care is an approach to a person's care that improves the quality of their life, and that of their carer and family, when they are living with advanced and progressive illness. The term 'palliative' is derived from the Latin word 'pallium', which means 'cloak or cover'; in palliative care a person's symptoms are not cured but 'cloaked' or minimised, through effective symptom management. The aim is to promote comfort, without cure, and to achieve a good quality of life. Chapter 5 of this book discusses the use of the nursing process in symptom management; the same principles should be applied when managing symptoms in palliative care. Quality of life is improved through the early identification of problems and the accurate assessment and treatment of them. Problems may be physical (e.g. pain), psychological (e.g. fear), social (e.g. stigma) and spiritual (e.g. loss of meaning). The World Health Organization (WHO, 2002, page 84) states that palliative care:

- provides relief from pain and other distressing symptoms;
- affirms life and regards dying as a natural process;
- intends neither to hasten or postpone death;
- integrates the psychosocial and spiritual aspects of patient care;
- offers a support system to help patients live as actively as possible until death;
- offers a support system to help the family cope during the patient's illness and in their own bereavement;
- uses a team approach to address the needs of patients and their families, including bereavement counselling, if indicated;
- will enhance quality of life, and may also positively influence the course of illness;
- is applicable early in the course of illness, in conjunction with other therapies that are intended to prolong life, such as chemotherapy or radiation therapy, and includes those investigations needed to better understand and manage distressing clinical complications.

Given that the disease progression of different LTCs varies – some people experience a sudden decline, others experience both a gradual decline and acute episodes and some have a steady yet progressive decline – it is important to view palliative care as part of the continuum of care a person living with an LTC receives. Palliative care should run alongside active management and be seen as ensuring quality of life at all stages of a person's life when they are living with an LTC. There should be no sudden shift from active management to palliative care; instead a transition process should be in place. As a person's LTC progresses and their symptoms increase, treatment that is aimed at modifying the LTC decreases, and at this point palliative care increases, providing support for the person and their carer and family before, during and after the person's death (WAG, 2003; DH, 2008e; TSG, 2008; DHSSPS, 2009).

Activity 7.3   *Evidence-based practice and research*

Palliative care is one of the terms used when discussing the care provision for people nearing the end of their life and describes an approach to a person's care. Other terms such as terminal care and supportive care can also be used to describe aspects of palliative care. Using available resources define the following:

- terminal care;
- supportive care.

Some useful resources:

DH (2008e) *End of Life Care Strategy: Promoting High Quality Care for All Adults at the End of Life.* London: DH.

National Institute for Clinical Excellence (NICE) (2004) *Improving Supportive and Palliative Care for Adults with Cancer: The Manual.* London: NICE.

A brief outline answer is given at the end of this chapter.

As you can see from Activity 7.3, terminal care and supportive care are aspects of palliative care. The term palliative care will be used throughout this chapter to mean care that is delivered in the end stages of a person's life but will incorporate aspects of the terms outlined in Activity 7.3. Palliative care is not delivered in a specific care setting; it can be delivered in a number of settings, e.g. a person's own home, nursing home or a hospice. Neither is it provided by one specific group of healthcare professionals: it is provided by many, including Macmillan nurses, district nurses, GPs and healthcare professionals working in secondary care.

The National End-of-life Care Strategy

This is an important strategy whose aim is to raise the profile of end-of-life care through the promotion of effective palliative care (DH, 2008e). The National EoLC strategy stated that there was a need to plan and deliver high quality services to ensure that people receiving palliative care would be able to choose where they were cared for and where they died (DH, 2008e). It also intended to reduce the number of emergency admissions of those who had expressly stated their wish to die at home and to decrease the number of older people admitted to a hospital setting from a residential/nursing home in the last week of their life. EoLC is an approach to care that allows the person to be treated as an individual, to receive effective symptom control and to die in the place of their choice with their family around them. Initiatives such as the Gold Standards Framework (GSF), preferred place, now priorities, of care (PPC) and advance care planning (ACP) are central to its success.

The Gold Standards Framework

The GSF is a UK-wide approach that can be used to support you to deliver effective palliative care in a primary care setting. You can apply the GSF approach to any person, in any setting; it focuses on enabling people to live well in the last years, months or days of their life (Thomas, 2003). The main focus of the GSF is to enable you, as part of a primary healthcare team, to work collaboratively to maximise a person's continuity of care, introduce ACP, promote symptom control and provide ongoing support. Through the use of GP practice based palliative care registers, linked in to the Quality Outcome Framework, those receiving palliative care are easily identified to all members of the practice team, improving communication and the care received. Both the GSF and the palliative care register promote the use of regular team meetings to discuss the needs of those on the palliative care register (DH, 2008e). The GSF will be discussed further in this chapter in the section on delivering holistic palliative care; the web link for the GSF website can be found in the useful websites section at the end of this chapter.

Preferred priorities of care

In 2003 Higginson, on behalf of the National Council for Palliative Care (NCPC), undertook a study into preferred place of death in the general population (Higginson, 2003). 56% of the respondents in this study stated that they would prefer to die at home. However, Holdsworth and Fisher (2010) argue that basing figures on healthy people may not be a true reflection of what actually occurs, especially if the lead up to a person's death is sudden or particularly challenging to manage. In their study of 298 hospice patients Holdsworth and Fisher (2010) found that only 26.8% stated a preference to die at home. It could be said that whether the number of people expressing a preference to die at home stands at 56% or 26.8% is irrelevant. What is important is that people are able to discuss their preferences and are supported to die in the place of their choice. Currently, however, this does not happen, with up to 58% of deaths in England taking place in an NHS hospital (DH, 2008e). To address this challenge as part of the EoLC strategy advance care planning was introduced, and the preferred priorities of care (PPC) document is an example of this.

Completing a PPC is a voluntary process. The completed document is kept by the person receiving palliative care, and the information on the PPC is shared with those planning and delivering their care. It documents aspects of their future care that is important to them, such as 'where would you like to be cared for in the future?' and 'what are your priorities for your future care?' and focuses on the person's beliefs and values. You can then use this information to ensure that the care you deliver takes into account what is important to that person. Relevant information from the PCC can also be used in future care planning. This is particularly useful should a person receiving palliative care no longer be able to make decisions themselves, e.g.

a person with dementia or a degenerative neurological condition. It should not be used to record information relating to refusal of medical treatment, as the PPC is not a legally binding document. You should endeavour to ensure that a person keeps their PCC up to date as their wishes and views may change over time (National EoLC, 2009). For those living with dementia or a degenerative neurological condition, who lack mental capacity, it may be necessary to discuss having a lasting power of attorney (LPA). An LPA is a document that allows a person living with an LTC to choose someone to make decisions on their behalf when they lack the mental capacity to do so themselves. Within the UK there may be slight variations in law as it relates to LPA and mental capacity, therefore you will need to familiarise yourself with the law as it relates to mental capacity and LPA in the country where you work.

Advance care planning (ACP)

ACP is a key component of the National EoLC strategy; it is a voluntary process that allows for an open discussion between the person receiving palliative care and those caring for them, including their family and carer. ACP differs from traditional care planning, which addresses current areas of need, such as reduced nutritional intake and how they are to be managed. ACP addresses a person's anticipated deterioration and what their preferences for treatment would be; this is especially relevant should the person's ability to communicate reduce or their capacity to make decisions deteriorates. The purpose of the discussion is to discuss and document the following (DH, 2008f):

- the person's wishes and concerns;
- the person's values and beliefs;
- the person's understanding of their condition and likely prognosis;
- the person's preferences for the type of care that may be appropriate as part of their future care.

It is important that any discussions you have are documented, reviewed regularly and communicated to appropriate people, including the person's carer and family, if required. Within the ACP framework there are two ways in which a person can state their preferences regarding their future care and management; these are (1) a statement of wishes and preferences, and (2) an advance decision to refuse treatment. Before discussing either of these options with a person in your care it is essential that you have an understanding of mental capacity and its relevance to ACP. Within the UK there may be slight variations in law as it relates to ACP and mental capacity, therefore you will need to familiarise yourself with the law as it relates to mental capacity and ACP in the country where you work.

Statement of wishes and preferences

A statement of wishes and preferences allows the person living with an LTC, who is in the palliative stages of their illness, to either write down or verbally express, and have documented, their wishes and preferences in relation to future treatment. This may take the form of explaining their feelings, beliefs and values that influence how they make decisions. It may also include areas of a person's care such as where they would like to be cared for, and what types of treatment they are prepared to have. While this is not a legally binding document, it does have legal standing as part of the Mental Capacity Act (MCA, 2005) and should be taken into account when deciding on a person's future treatment options.

Advance decision to refuse treatment

Some people living with an LTC may have strong feelings about specific treatments they would not want to have. In order to have this recognised it is necessary for an advance decision to refuse treatment (an Advance Directive) to be made. An advance decision to refuse treatment is a legally binding document and is part of the MCA (2005) and should only be made under the guidance of a healthcare professional who understands the process. It only applies if the person making the decision is over the age of 18 and has the mental capacity to make the necessary decision and will only come into effect if the person loses their capacity to make decisions about their treatment. An advance decision to refuse treatment allows the person to specifically express, and have documented, the type of medical treatment they wish to refuse, e.g. being treated with antibiotics for a chest infection. It must relate to specific treatments and circumstances and will only come into effect at these times (DH, 2008f).

ACP is a voluntary process that should be initiated by the person receiving the care. It should be handled sensitively and by a healthcare professional who has a clear understanding of the legal and ethical issues involved. The aspects of the EoLC strategy outlined above are there to support you in your delivery of appropriate and effective palliative care to people living with an LTC. Regardless of whether the person you are caring for has made explicit their preferences for care, ensuring that they are assessed correctly and that the care delivered meets their needs is your priority.

Holistic palliative care in long term conditions

Palliative care is delivered by a variety of healthcare professionals in a variety of settings. The NCPC state that palliative care can be provided by both generalist and specialist healthcare professionals. Generalists should be able to provide the day-to-day care for people requiring palliative care, their carer and family through effective assessment, management and appropriate referral to specialist services. Specialists, such as palliative care consultants and clinical nurse specialists, are healthcare professionals with a high level of knowledge and skill in the field of palliative care who are responsible for directing a plan of care that allows for the integration of available resources and services. This may include providing care and management in the person's home or in a local hospice, and bereavement support (NCPC, 2009).

Assessing for holistic palliative care

To enable both generalists and specialists to provide coordinated care to the person requiring palliative care and their family, it is important to fully assess the person and their needs. The End of Life Care Programme (EoLCP) has recently published guidance on how to assess the needs of a person requiring palliative care (EoLCP, 2010). This guidance will provide you with relevant information that will enable you to undertake a holistic assessment. The areas assessed are similar to the PEPSICOLA approach recommended by the GSF (Thomas, 2003). Whether you use the EoLCP holistic common assessment or the PEPSICOLA framework it is important that your assessment is holistic. Table 7.2 applies the PEPSICOLA approach to Mary, one of the scenarios you have been following in this book.

> ### Case study: Mary (see website: **www.learningmatters.co.uk/nursing** for full case study)
>
> *Mary was diagnosed with lung cancer after several months of increasing dyspnoea and dysphagia. Following her diagnosis she was offered a course of chemotherapy; however, following her first dose she developed **pancytopenia** and was admitted to hospital. Following this she declined any further chemotherapy. A course of radiotherapy followed with little improvement in her dyspnoea and dysphagia. A sudden deterioration due to a chest infection, from which she recovered slightly, and the realisation that her health was deteriorating prompted Mary to discuss end-of-life care issues with her family and GP.*

	Consider	Application to Mary
P — physical	• Assessment of symptoms, including pain chart • Overall management plan • Medication, both regular and PRN • Stopping non-essential treatment and medication • Treatment and medication side-effects	Mary is taking the following regular medication to manage her symptoms: MST 30 mg twice a day, oromorph 2.5 mg four hourly, domperidone 10 mg three times a day, diazepam 2 mg twice a day, lorazepam 1mg at night and lactulose 15 mg three times a day. She has a dosette box that her husband fills up; he also helps her to take her medication. Mary has decided not to have any further treatment for her lung cancer. Since her chest infection Mary has had oxygen at home; she uses this after exertion, e.g. moving from bed to commode. *continued opposite...*

Table 7.2:

continued...

E E – emotional	• What do they know about their illness? • What is their emotional reaction to their diagnosis? • How are family and friends coping? • Are there signs of clinical depression? • Do they have any dependents? • What signifies a deterioration, what to expect?	Mary is quite philosophical about her diagnosis and has tried to remain positive. She is aware that she is going to die and has discussed this with James and their children. Mary has many friends and has been able to, until recently, keep in touch with them via email. She has many visitors to the house, though due to her fatigue has to pace herself. James is coping extremely well with the situation and would like Mary to die at home. He does not talk much about how he is feeling, preferring to concentrate on the practical aspects of caring for Mary. Since her chest infection Mary has been quite clear that she does not want to go into hospital. She has spoken to her GP about this, who has recorded this on her notes and made this information available to the out-of-hours (OOH) service.
P P – personal	• Cultural background, language, sexuality, spiritual and religious needs	Mary has no strong religious beliefs and has asked for a humanist celebration of her life. Recently she met with the humanist celebrant to discuss some aspects of this, and now this is done she does not wish to talk about it further. She has made some notes about music. Mary wants to maintain her dignity throughout her illness.

continued overleaf...

	• **Consider**	**Application to Mary**
S — social support	• Social care assessment – have all appropriate benefits been claimed • Carer assessment • What aids are required? • What is the person's preferred place of care?	Due to their income Mary and James are not due any benefits. She has a disability badge for when she is out in the car. James does not want to draw attention to himself; the GP talks to him when he is here and has said to contact him if he needs anything. Mary has a hospital bed at home, two commodes (one with wheels and one without) and a perching stool. Mary has carers in to help with personal hygiene in the morning; at all other times James assists her. Mary, James and the family would like Mary to be cared for at home.
I — information and communication	• From person and their family to the primary healthcare team (PHCT) and vice versa • Communication between members of the PHCT • Patient held records • Communication – is person aware of plans and do they understand them? • Is communication appropriate?	Mary's case notes are kept at home and are easily accessible to healthcare professionals, Mary, James and their children. Relevant contact numbers are clearly identified on Mary's notes, e.g. who to contact during OOH. At all times since her diagnosis, Mary's GP has been open and honest and has consulted Mary on all aspects of her care. Relevant information has been provided to Mary in relation to her reduced oral intake, encouraging high protein supplements, etc. The GP and district nurses responsible for Mary's care discuss her condition on a daily basis; they are based in the same surgery and are able to discuss any issues that arise easily. They are also in contact with the Macmillan specialist nurse at the local hospital.

continued opposite...

continued...

C — control and autonomy	Level of need assess: • mental capacity • treatment options • preferred place (priority) of care • advance care planning • is there any conflict between the wishes of the person and the carer?	At the time of her diagnosis Mary wrote up her advance directive. A copy of this is held with her solicitor and her GP. All those involved in her care know that it is Mary's wish, and her family's wish, that she die at home. All members of the PHCT are supportive of this and are working to ensure that this is what happens.
O — out of hours	• Communication – between members of the PHCT and out of hours, does the person know what to do in an emergency? • Carer support – are night sitters needed? Provide written information • Medical support – document anticipated management • Medication	Mary's GP has ensured that OOH services are aware of her by using a handover form; this documents any anticipated needs to enable the out-of-hours service to respond appropriately. Mary and James have been offered a Marie Curie night sitter; however, they do not feel that this is necessary at the moment.
L — late	End-of-life/terminal care (last two days): • Is the person comfortable with good symptom control? • Are the person and their family aware of the situation? • Has all non-essential medication been stopped?	Mary is not yet in the last few days of her life. However, as there has been evidence of open communication between Mary, her family and the PHCT, it can be assumed that when the time comes this aspect of her care will be approached sensitively. Mary and her family know that she is going to die as a result of her lung cancer and that it is only going to be a matter of time.
A — after care	• Planning for bereavement • Provide information to family • Inform other members of the PHCT of the death	Mary has discussed her funeral requirements and has met with the humanist celebrant who will lead her funeral.

Table 7.2: PEPSICOLA holistic assessment (Thomas, 2003) applied to Mary

Case study: Andrew (see website: **www.learningmatters.co.uk/nursing** for full case scenario)

Despite trying to improve both his levels of exercise and his nutritional intake, Andrew's condition has continued to deteriorate. He has continued to have recurrent chest infections that have reduced his appetite further, increased his level of dyspnoea and drastically reduced his exercise tolerance. Since his last chest infection he has required **long term oxygen therapy** (LTOT) at home due to reduced oxygen saturation levels. David (Andrew's community matron) has graded his dyspnoea at 4 on the Medical Research Council dyspnoea scale. This indicates that Andrew has to stop for breath after walking about 100 metres or after a few minutes on level ground. His most recent **spirometry** result stated that his FEV1 (forced expired volume) was 30%, indicating end-stage COPD. Both Andrew's GP and David are concerned about his deteriorating condition and have asked each other the 'surprise' question: 'Would you be surprised if this person were to die in the next 6–12 months?' They both answered no to this question (Royal College of General Practitioners, 2008).

With the consent of his GP, David has discussed the results of Andrew's spirometry with him, and what this means for his future care with the emphasis being on palliative care. Andrew has said he would like to stay in his flat for as long as possible. However, he is now requiring homecare assistance in the morning and evening to assist him with his personal hygiene. He has meals on wheels five days of the week and a neighbour in the sheltered housing cooks a meal for him at the weekend. He is finding the change in his situation rather lonely as he is not able to get out and about. He has begun to talk about his wife Elizabeth recently.

Using the above information and accessing the full case scenario in the appendix, use the PEPSICOLA framework to assess Andrew's needs in relation to his palliative care.

A brief outline answer is given at the end of this chapter.

Having used the PEPSICOLA framework to assess Andrew's needs (Activity 7.3), and using the nursing process, you are now able to plan and implement an appropriate plan of care that will address his ongoing healthcare needs. Whatever a person's palliative care needs are, what is essential is that through effective communication and collaboration the person and their family receive the best care, by the most appropriate person in the place of their choice.

Delivering holistic palliative care

The GSF incorporates seven standards of care that relate to the effective delivery of holistic palliative care for people living with an LTC. Emphasis is placed on both direct care and management and the management and coordination of the healthcare professionals delivering the care (Thomas, 2003). Table 7.3 outlines these standards and their aims.

GSF standards of care	Aim and areas to consider
Communication	The aim of this standard is to improve *how* information is communicated, written, verbal and electronic, and *who* is involved in any communication, person receiving palliative care, out of hours, family, etc. A supportive care register allows a GP practice to record, monitor and review the care received by people in the last 6–12 months of their life. Through the use of monthly meetings proactive care and management can be planned, with ACP being incorporated if required.
Coordination	The aim of this standard is to ensure that the care delivered to people requiring palliative care is well organised and coordinated with communication being maintained. Each PHCT should have a nominated palliative care coordinator, e.g., practice nurse, district nurse. The palliative care coordinator is responsible for maintaining relevant paperwork, including the supportive care register, arranging the monthly meetings and ensuring appropriate tools such as PEPSICOLA are used.
Control of symptoms	The aim of this standard is to promote effective symptom management through the use of appropriate assessment such as PEPSICOLA. Each person receiving palliative care is assured of having a holistic assessment with the results being discussed and an appropriate person-centred plan of care being devised.
Continuity	The aim of this standard is to ensure continuity of care during out-of-hours, ensuring that the person receiving palliative care is supported during out-of-hours. Using the protocol devised by Calderdale and Kirklees Health Authority (Thomas, 2003) will promote continuity of care. It addresses four key areas: • communication – between GP/district nurse and out-of-hours service; • carer support – does the carer know what to do in a crisis, is a night sitter required? • medical support – any anticipated management documented in handover form; • drugs/equipment – leave any anticipated medication in person's home.

continued overleaf...

GSF standards of care	Aim and areas to consider
Continued learning	The aim of this standard is to promote reflective learning or 'learning as you go' to further develop the care given to people receiving palliative care. Through the use of practice-based teaching, significant event analysis and other learning opportunities, the professional development of those caring for people requiring palliative care is enhanced. Learning should focus on all areas of palliative care, strategic (planning of resources/coordination of services), clinical (treatment/management options) and personal (communication skills).
Carer support	The aim of this standard is to improve carer support: carers are key in enabling people receiving palliative care to remain in their own home. Through the provision of emotional and practical support carers are empowered to play as active a part as they would like to. Carer support does not stop when the person dies: bereavement support should be offered.
Care of the dying (terminal phase)	The aim of this standard is to promote suitable care in the last days of a person's life. Using such tools as the Liverpool Care Pathway for the Dying Patient will ensure that non-essential treatment is stopped, the person's symptoms are controlled and psychological and religious/spiritual support is available.

Table 7.3: The 7C's of the GSF (based on the work of Thomas, 2003)

Chapter summary

This chapter has provided you with an overview of breaking bad news, palliative care and the EoLC strategy. These important areas are all key aspects of the care and management of people living with an LTC. It has outlined some approaches that can be used when breaking bad news and applied these to your clinical practice. Palliative care and the EoLC strategy have been outlined in relation to providing appropriate care for people living with an LTC. Finally the importance of undertaking a holistic assessment has been discussed and applied to your clinical practice.

Having read through this chapter and undertaken the activities, you will have developed your knowledge and skills in relation to the principles of breaking bad news, palliative care, the EoLC strategy and how to assess a person's holistic palliative care needs. How you use the information in this chapter will depend on where you are working and your current roles and responsibilities. However, as a nurse, you can ensure that planning

continued overleaf...

continued...

for palliative care becomes part of your overall care and management of people living with an LTC. By having an increased awareness of some of the approaches that can be used when breaking bad news you will be better able to answer awkward questions and support those in your care. Increasing your knowledge of palliative care and the EoLC strategy will allow you to provide appropriate and relevant information to both the person living with an LTC and their carer, allowing them to make informed choices. Using frameworks such as PEPSICOLA will promote the delivery of person-centred holistic care that meets the ongoing needs of the person, their carer and family.

Activities: brief outline answers

Activity 7.3: Evidence-based practice and research (page 138)

- Terminal care – this is the care delivered to a person and their family in the last few months, weeks or days of their life. It focuses on addressing the needs of the person and their family that may become more important as death approaches. This might include preparing the person and the family for the death, supporting decision-making – preparing for when the person may not be able to make their own decisions – and ensuring that the person is comfortable.
- Supportive care – this is the care that assists the person and their family to cope with their condition from the point of diagnosis through to death and bereavement. It enables the person to maximise the benefits of any treatment, to improve the quality of life and should be given the same priority as active treatment. Supportive care is based on the premise that people diagnosed with cancer, or entering the palliative stages of an LTC, require care that supports them to make appropriate decisions and addresses their needs holistically. Supportive care can be delivered by both generalist and specialist healthcare professionals; it will also be delivered by the person's carer, family and friends.

Activity 7.4: Critical thinking (page 146)

P – physical	Review of Andrew's medication, use of bronchodilators and inhaled corticosteroids. Ongoing LTOT assessment and review: ensure Andrew is aware of the health and safety issues. Comprehensive assessment regarding other possible symptoms, e.g. pain, nutritional intake.
E – emotional	Having spoken to his community matron, Andrew is aware that his condition has deteriorated. He is concerned about being on his own as he is no longer able to get out and about as much as he could. Andrew has started talking about his wife Elizabeth recently; this may mean he is beginning to think about his own death. It is essential that Andrew knows who and how to contact people should his condition deteriorate. If he does not have one then a pendant alarm would be appropriate.
P – personal	We don't know a lot about Andrew's personal beliefs; this is the time to begin to discuss these with him. It may be useful to find out what kind of funeral service he arranged for Elizabeth.

continued overleaf...

continued...

S – social support	Is Andrew claiming all the available benefits; has a DS1500 been completed? Social isolation is a potential problem; Andrew enjoys company but may become increasingly isolated due to his dyspnoea. Does he have all the necessary aids at home to promote his independence? Andrew has indicated that he would like to stay in his flat for as long as possible; how to manage this and alternatives may have to be discussed.
I – information and communication	Does Andrew hold a copy of his case notes; are they accessible to all relevant members of the PHCT? Andrew has a community matron; does he know how to contact her? Andrew is aware that his condition is deteriorating, and it may be appropriate to discuss issues such as his will with him.
C – control and autonomy	We do not know what Andrew's thoughts are on his future care apart from the fact that he would like to stay in his flat for as long as possible. It is necessary to discuss preferred place of care and advance directives with him to ensure that his wishes are met.
O – out of hours	Communication between the community matron, GP and OOH service should ensure that all know what to do in the case of a deterioration in Andrew's conditions. Andrew should know who and how to contact the out-of-hours service.
L – late	Not yet applicable – though through effective communication and working in partnership with Andrew when the time comes, end-of-life issues should be able to be discussed to ensure appropriate care.
A – after	This may not be discussed, though allowing Andrew time to talk about Elizabeth and her death you may be able to talk to Andrew about his own funeral.

Further reading

Greenstreet, W (2004) Why nurses need to understand the principles of bereavement theory. *British Journal of Nursing*, 13(10): 590–93.
This article provides a review of the most well known bereavement models.

McEnhill, L S (2008) Breaking bad news of cancer to people with learning disabilities. *British Journal of Learning Disabilities*, 36: 157–64.
This is an interesting article that applies the SPIKES 6 step protocol to meeting the needs of people with a learning disability when breaking bad news.

NHS End-of-life Care Programme and the National Council for Palliative Care (2008) *Advance Decisions to Refuse Treatment, a Guide for Health and Social Care Professionals.* 10350. Leicester: End-of-life Care Programme.
A comprehensive guide to understanding the MCA as it relates to advance decisions to refuse treatment.

Thomas, K (2003) *Caring for the Dying at Home: Companions on the Journey.* Abingdon: Radcliffe Publishing.
This is the official textbook of the Gold Standards Framework (GSF), and supports and allows those working in primary care to make improvements in the care they give to people nearing the end of their life.

Useful websites

www.act.org.uk
This is the website for the Association for Children with Life-Threatening Illnesses (ACT). It is a UK-wide charity whose focus is on ensuring that children and young people living with a life-threatening illness receive the best quality care.

www.endoflifecareforadults.nhs.uk
This is the website for the National End of Life Care Programme, and contains relevant information relating to end-of-life care and includes useful case studies.

www.goldstandardsframework.nhs.uk
This is a UK-wide framework aimed at enabling generalists to maximise the care they deliver to people nearing the end of their life. This website provides information regarding all aspects of the GSF, including how to use it in a variety of settings, e.g. continuing care, secondary care, available research and the GSF toolkit.

www.ncpc.org.uk
The National Council for Palliative Care (NCPC) is an umbrella organisation for all those involved in providing, commissioning and using palliative care services in England, Wales and Northern Ireland. Its aim is to promote palliative care for all who need it. This site contains useful information on all aspects of palliative care, including publications.

www.palliativecarescotland.org.uk
This organisation has the same remit as the NCPC but in Scotland; it supports and contributes to the strategic direction of palliative care in Scotland. This site contains information on all aspects of their work, including publications.

www.pallium.ca
This is the website for a Canadian palliative care project; there is a video library that uses dramatisation to explore palliative care issues such as breaking bad news.

Glossary

Atonic: lacking in normal muscle tone

Atopy: a genetic tendency that predisposes a person to develop a hypersensitive response to common environmental allergens, for example, asthma, eczema, hay fever

Autonomy: when a person is able to make decisions about, and take responsibility for, their own situation

Bullae: a large blister or vesicle

Clonic: an abnormal neuromuscular activity resulting in alternating muscle relaxation and contraction, for example, tonic–clonic epileptic seizure

Comorbidity: the presence of one or more diseases and the effect of these diseases on the person

Compliance: agreement and cooperation, for example, a person taking their medication as prescribed

Concordance: agreement to participate in something, for example, concordance with medication regime, i.e., a person agreeing with the prescriber to take their prescribed medication as directed

Continuous ambulatory peritoneal dialysis (CAPD): renal dialysis that takes place inside the person's body using their peritoneum as the dialysis membrane; this form of dialysis is done at home, usually four times a day, and takes approximately 30 minutes each time

Determinants of health: these are the factors that affect a person's health and include the person's social and economic environment, the person's physical environment and the person's individual characteristics and behaviour

Distal: situated away from the point of origin or attachment

Emotional intelligence: awareness of your own emotions and those of others

Enabling: to assist a person to become able to do something, to make something possible

Epidemiology: the study of the occurrence, transmission and control of infectious diseases, for example, tuberculosis

Estimated glomerular filtration rate (eGFR): this test estimates the volume of blood that is filtered by the kidneys over a set period of time. The test measures the level of creatinine in the blood; if levels are elevated this indicates that the kidneys are not working as efficiently as they should

Ethos: the fundamental character or spirit that defines a belief, person, group or community

Hyperplasia: an abnormal increase in cell number

Hypertrophy: an abnormal increase in the cell size

Long term oxygen therapy (LTOT): oxygen therapy that is usually delivered for a minimum of 15 hours per day, including overnight; once this is started it is likely that a person will be on this for the rest of their life

Orthopnea: difficulty in breathing when lying down; it is usually relieved when the person sits or stands up

Osmolality: a measurement of concentration in a liquid that moves through a semi-permeable membrane

Pancytopenia: a reduction in the number of red blood cells, white blood cells and platelets

Philosophy: the rationale investigation of the truths and principles of reality, knowledge and ethics.

Polyneuropathy: a disorder that affects peripheral nerves, which can result in a person experiencing reduced sensation, for example, reduced ability to detect heat

Primary care: care delivered in or close to a person's home, for example, general practitioner practices, NHS walk-in centres and pharmacists

Prizing: to demonstrate that you value and respect someone

Public health: the area of health concerned with the promotion of health and the reduction of health inequalities in the population; it includes the physical, social, mental and economic health of the population

QoL: abbreviation for quality of life

Respite care: short term temporary care that is arranged to provide a break for those caring for people living with an LTC, for example, residential respite (where nursing or residential care is provided) or domiciliary respite (where care is provided in the person's own home)

Secondary care: medical services and hospital care, including elective and emergency care; access is often via a referral from primary care

Self-efficacy: a person's belief that they can make a change to their current situation

Spirometry: a test that determines the breathing capacity of the lungs; it measures both the forced vital capacity (the volume of air expired until a person feels their lungs are empty) and the forced expired volume (the volume of air expired in the first second of expiration)

Status asthmaticus: repeated asthma attacks, without relief, that do not respond to treatment

Syndrome: disease that has a distinct pattern of signs and symptoms, for example, dementia, Down's syndrome

Tertiary care: specialised care and treatment that is usually provided in specialist centres

Tonic: an increase in tone in a person's muscles, for example, contraction or convulsion

Transient: a condition that is temporary and usually lasts only a short time, for example, a transient ischaemic attack

References

Adler, R, Rosenfeld, L and Towne, N (1989) *Interplay: The Process of Interpersonal Communication.* Orlando, FL: Rinehart and Winston.

Alzheimer's Society (2009) *Counting the Cost: Caring for People with Dementia in Hospital Wards.* London: Alzheimer's Society.

Bach, S and Grant, A (2009) *Communication and Interpersonal Skills for Nurses.* Exeter: Learning Matters.

Baile, W F, Buckman, R, Lenzi, R, Glober, G, Beale, E A and Kudelka, A P (2000) SPIKES – A Six-Step Protocol for Delivering Bad News: Application to the Patient with Cancer. *The Oncologist,* 5: 302–11.

Barclay, M P, Cherry, D and Mittman, B S (2005) Improving Quality of Health Care for Dementia: A Consumer Approach. *Clinical Gerontologist,* 29 (2): 45–60.

Barker, P (2001) The tidal model: the lived-experience in person-centred mental health nursing care. *Nursing Philosophy,* 2: 213–23.

Barnes, S, Gott, M, Payne, S, Parker, C, Seamark, D, Gariballa, S and Small, N (2006) Characteristics and views of family carers of older people with heart failure. *International Journal of Palliative Nursing,* 12 (8): 380–89.

Barrett, D, Wilson, B and Woolands, A (2009) *Care Planning: A Guide for Nurses.* Harlow: Pearson Education Limited.

Bee, P E, Barnes, P and Luker, K A (2008) A systematic review of informal caregivers' needs in providing home-based end-of-life care to people with cancer. *Journal of Clinical Nursing,* 18: 1379–93.

Booth, K, Maguire, P M, Butterworth, T and Hillier, V F (1996) Perceived professional support and the user of blocking behaviours by hospice nurses. *Journal of Advanced Nursing,* 24: 522–27.

Boyd, S D (1998) Using active listening: improve your communication skills with the most powerful tool available. *Nursing Management,* July: 55.

Brewin, A (2004) The quality of life of carers of patients with severe lung disease. *British Journal of Nursing,* 13 (15): 906–12.

British Association of Enteral and Parenteral Nutrition (BAPEN) (2003) *The 'MUST' Explanatory Booklet: A Guide to the 'Malnutrition Universal Screening Tool' ('MUST') for Adults.* Redditch: BAPEN.

British National Formulary 60 (2010) *List of drug interaction: muscle relaxants* [online]. Available from http://bnf.org/bnf/bnf/current/41001i616.htm (registration to site required) [accessed: 23 November 2010].

British Thoracic Society and Scottish Intercollegiate Guidelines Network (2009) *British Guidelines on the Management of Asthma: A National Clinical Guideline* [online]. Available from www.sign.ac.uk/pdf/sign101. pdf [accessed: 20 October 2010].

Brooker, D and Duce, L (2000) Wellbeing and activity in dementia: a comparison group reminiscence therapy, structured goal-directed group activity and unstructured time. *Age and Mental Health,* 4 (4): 354–58.

Cancer Research UK (2010) *Prostate cancer risks and causes* [online]. Available from: www.cancerhelp.org. uk/type/prostate-cancer/about/prostate-cancer-risks-and-causes [accessed: 16 November 2010].

Care Services Improvement Partnership (2006) *Long-term Conditions and Depression: Considerations for Best Practice in Practice Based Commissioning.* Cheshire: Care Services Improvement Partnership.

Carers and Disabled Children Act 2000 [online]. Available from: www.legislation.gov.uk/ ukpga/2000/16/contents [accessed: 8 April 2011].

Carers (Equal Opportunities) Act 2004 [online]. Available from: www.legislation.gov.uk/ ukpga/2004/15/contents [accessed: 8 April 2011].

Carers (Recognition and Services) Act 1995 [online]. Available from: www.legislation.gov.uk/ ukpga/1995/12/contents [accessed: 8 April 2011].

Carers UK (2009) *Facts about caring* [online]. Available from: www.carersuk.org/Newsandcampaigns/ Media/Factsaboutcaring [accessed: 8 April 2011].

Caress, A L, Luker, K A, Chalmers, K I and Salmon, M P (2008) A review of the information and support needs of family carers of patients with chronic obstructive pulmonary disease. *Journal of Clinical Nursing*, 18: 479–91.

Carmichael, F and Hulme, C (2008) Are the needs of carers being met? *Journal of Community Nursing*, 22 (8/9): 4–12.

Carrier, J (2009) *Managing Long-term Conditions and Chronic Illness in Primary Care: A Guide to Good Practice.* Abindon: Routledge.

Chamber, M and Ryan, A A (2001) Exploring the emotional support needs and coping strategies of family carers. *Journal of Psychiatric and Mental Health Nursing*, 8: 99–106.

Cherniss, C (1998) *A Technical Report on Emotional Intelligence in Organisations.* The Consortium for Research on Emotional Intelligence in Organizations: USA. www.eiconsortium.org

Chilton, S, Melling, K, Drew, D and Clarridge A (2004) *Nursing in the Community: An Essential Guide to Practice.* London: Hodder Arnold.

Christensen, M and Hewitt-Taylor, J (2006) Empowerment in nursing: paternalism or maternalism? *British Journal of Nursing*, 15 (13): 695–99.

Chronic Pain Policy Coalition (2007) *A New Pain Manifesto* [online]. Available from: www.policyconnect. org/cppc/our-campaign [accessed: 8 April 2011].

Clark, D (2002) Between hope and acceptance: The medicalisation of dying. *British Medical Journal*, 324: 7342.905–07.

Clinical Knowledge Summaries (2005) *Urological cancer – suspected* [online]. Available from: www.cks. nhs.uk/urological_cancer_suspected/management/scenario_urological_cancer_suspected/prostate_ cancer#394927001 [accessed: 16 November 2010].

Clinical Knowledge Summaries (2007) *Asthma* [online]. Available from: www.cks.nhs.uk/asthma/ background_information/definition#297035001 [accessed: 16 November 2010].

Clinical Knowledge Summaries (2009a) *Heart failure – Chronic* [online]. Available from: www.cks.nhs.uk/ heart_failure_chronic#375288001 [accessed: 16 November 2010].

Clinical Knowledge Summaries (2009b) *Epilepsy.* [online]. Available from: www.cks.nhs.uk/epilepsy #37528400 [accessed: 16 November 2010].

Clinical Knowledge Summaries (2009c) *Angina – Stable* [online]. Available from: www.cks.nhs.uk/angina/ evidence/references#385559001 [accessed: 8 April 2011].

Clinical Knowledge Summaries (2009d) *Rheumatoid Arthritis.* [online]. Available from: www.cks.nhs.uk/ rheumatoid_arthritis#375741001 [accessed: 8 April 2011].

Clinical Knowledge Summaries (2009e) *Parkinson's Disease* [online]. Available from: www.cks.nhs.uk/ parkinsons_disease#380211001 [accessed: 8 April 2011].

Clinical Knowledge Summaries (2010a) *HIV Infection and AIDS* [online]. Available from: www.cks.nhs.uk/hiv_infection_and_aids~398479001 [accessed: 16 November 2010].

Clinical Knowledge Summaries (2010b) *Dementia* [online]. Available from: www.cks.nhs.uk/dementia#406236001 [accessed: 17 November 2010].

Clinical Knowledge Summaries (no date) *Multiple Sclerosis* [online]. Available from: www.cks.nhs.uk/patient_information_leaflet/multiple_sclerosis#463786000 [accessed: 17 November 2010].

Clinical Knowledge Summaries (no date) *Diabetes, Type 1* [online]. Available from: www.cks.nhs.uk/patient_information_leaflet/diabetes_type_1 [accessed: 17 November 2010].

Cohen, R, Leis, A M, Kuhl, D, Charbonneau, C, Ritvo, P and Ashbury, F D (2006) QOLLTI-f: measuring family carer quality of life. *Palliative Medicine*, 20: 755–67.

Community Care and Health (Scotland) Act 2002 [online]. Available from: www.legislation.gov.uk/asp/2002/5/contents [accessed: 8 April 2011].

ContinYou (2010) *Skilled for Health* [online]. Available from: www.continyou.org.uk/health_and_well_being/skilled_health/ [accessed: 11 October 2010].

Cook, J B (1984) Reminiscing: how can it help confused nursing home residents? *Journal of Contemporary Social Work*, 65: 90–93.

Corben, S and Rosen, R (2005) *Self-management for Long-term Conditions: Patient's Perspectives on the Way Ahead.* London: King's Fund.

Department of Health (1999) *The National Service Framework for Mental Health: Modern Standards and Service Models.* London: Department of Health.

Department of Health (2000a) *The NHS Plan: A Plan for Investment, a Plan for Reform.* Cm4818-1. London: The Stationery Office.

Department of Health (2000b) *National Service Framework for Coronary Heart Disease.* London: Department of Health.

Department of Health (2001) *National Service Framework for Older People.* 23633. London: Department of Health.

Department of Health (2004) *The National Service Framework for Children, Young People and Maternity Services: Core Standards.* 3779. London: Department of Health.

Department of Health (2005a) *The National Service Framework for Long Term Conditions.* 265106. London: Department of Health.

Department of Health (2005b) *Supporting People with Long Term Conditions: An NHS and Social Care Model to Support Local Innovation and Integration.* 4230. London: Department of Health.

Department of Health (2005c) *Self Care – A Real Choice: Self Care Support – A Practical Option.* 266332. London: Department of Health.

Department of Health (2006a) *Transition: Getting it Right for Young People. Improving the Transition of Young People with Long Term Conditions from Children's to Adult Health Services.* 5914. London: Department of Health.

Department of Health (2006b) *Our Health, Our Care, Our Say: A New Direction for Community Services.* Cm 6737. London: Department of Health.

Department of Health (2007) *Generic Choice Model for Long Term Conditions.* 9198. London: Department of Health.

Department of Health (2008a) *High Quality Care For All: NHS Next Stage Review Final Report.* Cm 7432. London: The Stationery Office.

Department of Health (2008b) *Raising the Profile of Long Term Conditions Care: a Compendium of Information.* 8734. London: Department of Health.

Department of Health (2008c) *Improving the Health and Well-Being of People with Long Term Conditions: World Class Services for People with Long Term Conditions – Information Tool Kit for Commissioners.* 12121. London: Department of Health.

Department of Health (2008d) *Transition: Moving on Well.* 8651. London: Department of Health.

Department of Health (2008e) *End of Life Care Strategy: Promoting High Quality Care for All Adults at the End of Life.* London: Department of Health.

Department of Health (2008f) *Advance Care Planning: A Guide for Health and Social Care Staff.* 7793. London: Department of Health.

Department of Health (2009a) *Caring with Confidence* [online]. Available from: webarchive.national archives.gov.uk/+/www.dh.gov.uk/en/SocialCare/Carers/DH_075475 [accessed: 4 August 2010].

Department of Health (2009b) *Your Health, Your Way: A Guide to Long Term Conditions and Self Care.* 12934. London: Department of Health.

Department of Health. (2010a) *Equity and Excellence: Liberating the NHS.* Cm 7881. London: The Stationery Office.

Department of Health (2010b) *The NHS Quality, Innovation, Productivity and Prevention Challenge: An Introduction for Clinicians.* London: Department of Health.

Department of Health and Social Services (2007) *Designed to Improve Health and the Management of Chronic Conditions in Wales: An Integrated Model and Framework.* Cardiff: Welsh Assembly Government.

Department of Health, Social Services and Public Safety (2005) *Caring for People Beyond Tomorrow: A Strategic Framework for the Development of Primary Health and Social Care for Individuals, Families and Communities in Northern Ireland.* Belfast: DHSSPS.

Department of Health, Social Services and Public Safety (2006) *Caring for Carers: Recognising, Valuing and Supporting the Caring Role.* Belfast: DHSSPS.

Department of Health, Social Services and Public Safety (2009a) *Service Framework for Cardiovascular Health and Wellbeing.* Belfast: DHSSPS.

Department of Health, Social Services and Public Safety (2009b) *Service Framework for Respiratory Health and Wellbeing.* Belfast: DHSSPS.

Department of Health, Social Services and Public Safety (2009c) *Palliative and End of Life Care Strategy for Northern Ireland: Consultation Document.* Belfast: DHSSPS.

DiClemente, C C (2007) The Transtheoretical Model of Intentional Behaviour Change. *Drugs and Alcohol Today,* 7(1): 29–32.

Dixon, A (2008) *Motivation and Confidence: What Does it Take to Change Behaviour?* London: King's Fund.

Douglas-Dunbar, M and Gardiner, P (2007) Support for carers of people with dementia during hospital admission. *Nursing Older People,* 19 (8): 27–30.

Drennan, V and Goodman, C (eds) (2007) *Oxford Handbook of Primary Care and Community Nursing.* Oxford: Oxford University Press.

Employment Act 2008 .[online]. Available from: www.legislation.gov.uk/ukpga/2008/24/contents [accessed: 8 April 2011].

Endacott, R, Jevon, P and Cooper, S (eds) (2009) *Clinical Nursing Skills: Core and Advanced.* Oxford: Oxford University Press.

References

Epictetus (AD 55–*c*135) *We have two ears and one mouth so that we can listen twice as much as we speak* [online]. Available from: http://thinkexist.com/quotation/we_have_two_ears_and_one_mouth_so_that_we_can/7650.html [accessed: 8 April 2011].

Expert Patients Programme (2009) *Looking after Me* [online]. Available from: ww.expertpatients.co.uk/course-participants/courses/looking-after-me [accessed: 4 August 2010].

Felce, D, Baxter, H, Lowe, K, Dunstan, F, Houston, H, Jones, G, Felce, J and Kerr, M (2008) The Impact of Repeated Health Checks for Adults with Learning Disabilities. *Journal of Applied Research in Intellectual Disabilities,* Journal compilation. Oxford: Blackwell.

Fitzsimons, D, Mullan, D, Wilson, J S, Conway, B, Corcoran, B, Dempster, M, Gamble, J, Stewart, C Rafferty, S, McMahon, M, MacMahon, J, Mulholland, P, Stockdale, P, Chew, E, Hanna, L, Brown, J, Ferguson, G and Fogarty, D (2007) The Challenge of patients' unmet palliative care needs in the final stages of chronic illness. *Palliative Medicine,* 21: 313–22.

Flemming, E, Carter, B and Gillibrand, W (2002) The transition of adolescents with diabetes from the children's health service into the adult health care service: a review of the literature. *Journal of Clinical Nursing,* 11: 560–67.

Foster, T and Hawkins, J (2005). The therapeutic relationship: dead or merely impeded by technology? *British Journal of Nursing,* 14 (13): 698–702.

Freshwater, D and Stickley, T J (2004) The heart of the art: emotional intelligence in nurse education. *Nursing Inquiry,* 11: 2.91–98.

Friedman, R and James, J W (2008) The Myth of the Stages of Dying, Death and Grief. *Skeptic,* 14: 2.37–41.

Gardener, H (1983, 1993) *Frames of Mind: The Multiple Intelligences.* New York: Basic Books (second edition published in Britain by Fontana Press).

Gardner, H (1999) *Intelligence Reframes. Multiple Intelligences for the 21st Century.* New York: Basic Books.

General Medical Council (2006) *Good Medical Practice* [online]. Available from: www.gmc-uk.org/guidance/good_medical_practice.asp [accessed: 5 August 2010].

Gibbs, G (1988) *Learning by Doing: A Guide to Teaching and Learning Methods.* Oxford: Further Education Unit, Oxford Brookes University.

Gibson, P G and Powell, H (2004) Written action plans for asthma: an evidence-based review of the key components. *Thorax,* 59: 94–99.

Gray, E (2004) The management of pain in multiple sclerosis: a care-study approach. *British Journal of Nursing,* 13 (17): 1017–20.

Greenhalgh, T and Hurwitz, B (1999) Narrative Based Medicine: why study narrative? *British Medical Journal,* 318: 48–50.

Greer, S (1999) Mind-body research in psychooncology. *Advances in Mind-Body Medicine,* 15: 236–81.

Greer, S, Watson, M, Haviland, J, Davidson, J and Bliss, J (2000) Fighting spirit in patients with cancer. *The Lancet,* 4: 847.

Haddad, M (2010) Caring for patients with long-term conditions and depression. *Nursing Standard,* 24 (24): 40–49.

Heath, H (2010) Improving the quality of care for people with dementia in general hospitals. *Quality of Care Supplement,* 1–16.

Higginson, I (2003) *Priorities for End of Life Care in England, Wales and Scotland.* London: National Council for Palliative Care.

Hippocrates (460–370 BC) *Cure sometime: treat often: comfort always* [online]. Available from: www.searchquotes.com/quotation/Cure_sometimes,_treat_often,_comfort_always./118801/ [accessed: 8 April 2011].

Hippocratic Oath: Modern Version (1964) [online]. Available from: http://pbs.org/wgbh/nova/doctors/oath_modern.html [accessed: 8 April 2011].

Holdsworth, L and Fisher, S (2010) A retrospective analysis of preferred and actual place of death for hospice patients. *International Journal of Palliative Care,* 16 (9): 424–30.

Holman, H and Lorig, K (2002) Patients as partners in managing chronic disease. British *Medical Journal,* 302: 526–27.

Huang, S L, Li, C M, Yang, C Y and Chen, J J J (2009) Application of Reminiscence Treatment on Older People with Dementia: A Case Study in Pingtung, Taiwan. *Journal of Nursing Research,* 17 (2): 112–18.

Hutt, R, Rosen, R and McCauley, J (2004) *Case-Managing Long-Term Conditions: What Impact does it have in the Treatment of Older People?* London: The King's Fund.

International Association for the Study of Pain (1986) Classification of Chronic Pain, 34 (supplement 3): 51–226. In: Charlton, R (ed.) (2002) *Primary Palliative Care: Dying, Death and Bereavement in the Community.* Abingdon: Radcliffe Medical Press, p. 49.

Kaye, P (1996) *Breaking Bad News (Pocket Book).*Northampton: EPL Publications.

Kickbusch, I S (2001) Health literacy: addressing the health and education divide. *Health Promotion International,* 16 (3): 289–97.

Knight, J (2009) Songs for Learning. *Nursing Standard,* 23 (43): 22–23.

Kübler-Ross, E and Kessler, D (2005) *On Grief and Grieving: Finding the Meaning of Grief through the Five Stages of Loss.* London: Simon Schuster UK Ltd.

Kübler-Ross, E (2009) *On Death and Dying: What the Dying Have to Teach Doctors, Nurses, Clergy and their own Family,* 40th anniversary edition. Abingdon: Routledge.

Launer, J (2002) *Narrative-based Primary Care: A Practical Guide.* Abingdon: Radcliffe Medical Press.

Launer, J (2006), New Stories for Old: Narrative Based Primary Care in Great Britain. *Families, Systems and Health,* 24 (3): 336–44.

Lindsey, M (2002) Comprehensive health care services for people with learning disabilities. *Advances in Psychiatric Treatment,* 8: 138–47.

Long Term Conditions Alliance Northern Ireland (2008) *Response to Proposals for Health and Social Care Reform in Northern Ireland* [online]. Available from: www.ltcani.org.uk/resources/Response-NHS-reforms-May08.pdf [accessed: 4 August 2010].

Lorig, K, Holman, H, Sobel, D, Laurent, D, Gonzales, V and Minor, M (2006) *Living a Healthy Life with Chronic Conditions: Self-Management of Heart Disease, Arthritis, Diabetes, Asthma, Bronchitis, Emphysema and others.* Boulder: Bull Publishing Company.

Marmot Review (2010) *Fair Society, Healthy Lives: Strategic Review of Health Inequalities in England post-2010.* The Marmot Review. London: Department of Health and University College London.

Mason, P (2008) Motivational interviewing. *Practice Nurse,* 35 (3).

McGrath, A and Yeowart, C (2009) *Rights of Passage: Supporting Disabled Young People through the Transition to Adulthood.* London: New Philanthropy Capital.

McKenna, J (2007) Emotional intelligence training in adjustment to physical disability and illness. *International Journal of Therapy and Rehabilitation*, 14 (12): 551–56.

Mental Capacity Act (2005) [online]. Available from: www.legislation.gov.uk/ukpga/2005/9/contents [accessed: 8 April 2011].

Mezuk, B, Eaton, W W, Albrecht, S and Golden, S H (2008) Depression and type 2 diabetes over the lifespan: a meta analysis. *Diabetes Care*, 31 (12): 2383–90.

Middleton, S, Barnett, J and Reeves, D (2001) *What is an Integrated Pathway?* London: Hayward Medical Communications.

NHS Employers (2009) *Quality and Outcomes Framework Guidance for GMS Contract 2009/10: Delivering Investment in General Practice.* Leeds: NHS Employers.

Naidoo, J and Wills, J (2009) *Foundations for Health Promotion (Public Health and Health Promotion.* London: Baillière Tindall.

National Council for Palliative Care (2009) *Palliative Care Explained* [online]. Available at: www.ncpc.org. uk/palliative_care.html [accessed: 17 December 2010].

National End of Life Care Programme (2009) *Fact Sheet 5: Preferred Priorities for Care (PCC)* [online]. Available at: www.endoflifecareforadults.nhs.uk/publications/factsheet5 [accessed: 17 December 2010].

National End of Life Care Programme (2010) *Holistic Common Assessment of Supportive and Palliative Care Needs for Adults Requiring End of Life Care* [online]. Available at: www.endoflifecareforadults.nhs.uk/assets/downloads/HCA_guide.pdf [accessed: 14 December 2010].

National Institute for Clinical Excellence (2004) *Improving Supportive and Palliative Care for Adults with Cancer: The Manual.* London: NICE.

National Institute for Health and Clinical Excellence (2009a) *Depression in Adults with a Chronic Physical Health Problem: Treatment and Management.* London: NICE.

National Institute for Health and Clinical Excellence (2009b) *Depression: The Treatment and Management of Depression in Adults (partial update of NICE guideline 23).* London: NICE.

National Institute for Health and Clinical Excellence (2009c) *Rheumatoid Arthritis: The Management of Rheumatoid Arthritis in Adults.* London: NICE.

National Institute for Health and Clinical Excellence (2010) *Chronic Obstructive Pulmonary Disease: Management of Chronic Obstructive Pulmonary Disease in Adults in Primary and Secondary Care (partial update).* London: NICE.

National Prescribing Centre (2007a) *Patients and their Medicines* [online]. Available from: www.npci.org.uk/medicines_management/patients/patientsmed/resources/5mg_pm.pdf [accessed: 22 October 2010].

National Prescribing Centre (2007b) *Medicines Use Reviews* [online]. Available from: www.npci.org.uk/medicines_management/review/mediuse/resources/5mg_mur.pdf [accessed: 22 October 2010].

National Prescribing Centre (2007c) *Self Administration of Medicines* [online]. Available from: www.npci.org.uk/medicines_management/safety/selfadmin/resources/5mg_sam.pdf [accessed: 22 October 2010].

National Prescribing Centre (2010) *Non-medical Prescribing by Nurses, Optometrists, Pharmacists, Physiotherapists, Podiatrists and Radiographers: A Quick Guide for Commissioners.* Liverpool: National Prescribing Centre.

Nawate, Y, Kaneko, F, Hanaoka, H and Okamura, H (2008) Efficacy of Group Reminiscence Therapy for Elderly Dementia Patients Residing at Home: A Preliminary Report. *Physical & Occupational Therapy in Geriatrics*, 26 (3): 57–68.

NHS Institute for Innovation and Improvement (2010) *High Impact Actions for Nursing and Midwifery* [online]. Available from: www.institute.nhs.uk/building_capability/general/aims/ [accessed: 8 April 2011].

Nicholson, A, Kuper, H and Hemingway, H (2006) Depression as an aetiologic and prognostic factor in coronary heart disease: a meta-analysis of 6362 events among 146 538 participants in 54 observational studies. *European Heart Journal*, 27 (23): 2763–74.

Nursing and Midwifery Council (2008) *The Code: Standards of Conduct, Performance and Ethics for Nurses and Midwives.* London: Nursing and Midwifery Council.

Nursing and Midwifery Council (2010) *Standards for Pre-registration Nursing.* London: Nursing and Midwifery Council.

Nutbeam, D (2000) Health literacy as a public health goal: a challenge for contemporary health education and communication strategies into the 21st century. *Health Promotion International*, 15 (3): 259–67.

O'Baugh, J, Wilkes, L M, Luke, S and George, A (2003) 'Being positive': perceptions of patients with cancer and their nurses. *Journal of Advanced Nursing*, 44 (3): 262–70.

Offredy, M, Bunn, F and Morgan, J (2009) Case management in long term conditions: an inconsistent journey? *British Journal of Community Nursing*, 14 (6): 252–57.

Okomura, Y, Tanimukai, S and Asada, T (2008) Effects of short-term reminiscence therapy on elderly with dementia: A comparison with everyday conversation approaches. *Psychogeriatrics*, 8: 124–33.

Office of National Statistics (2009) *Life Expectancy in the United Kingdom: Female Life Expectancy 1992–2007, by Local Authority* [online]. Available from www.statistics.gov.uk/life-expectancy/lifemap.html [accessed: 7 October 2010].

Office of National Statistics (2010) *Population Estimates: UK population grows to 61.8 million* [online]. Available from: www.statistics.gov.uk/cci/nugget.asp?id=6 [accessed: 8 April 2011].

Orem, D E (1980) *Nursing: Concepts of Practice.* New York: McGraw Hill.

Papastravrou, E, Kalokerniou, A, Papacostas, S S, Tsangari, H and Sourtzi, P (2007) Caring for a Relative with Dementia: Family Caregiver Burden. *Journal of Advanced Nursing: Original Research, Journal Compilation.* Oxford: Blackwell Publishing Ltd.

Patel, H and Gwilt, C (2008) *Crash Course: Respiratory System.* Edinburgh: Mosby/Elsevier.

Patrick, D L and Erickson, P (1993) *Health Status and Health Policy: Quality of Life in Health Care Evaluation and Resource Allocation.* New York: Oxford University Press.

Phillips, J (2009) Improving access to self-management services. *British Journal of Neuroscience Nursing*, 5 (11): 524–25.

Porth, C M and Matfin, G (2010) *Essentials of Pathophysiology: Concepts of Altered Health Status (International Edition).* China: Wolters Kluwer Health/Lippincott: Williams and Wilkins.

Princess Royal Trust for Carers (2010) *The Princess Royal Trust for Carers 'Out of Hospital' Project – Learning from the Pilot Projects.* York: Acton Shapiro consultancy and research.

Radziewicz, R and Baile, W F (2001). Communication skills: Breaking bad news in the clinical setting. *Oncology Nursing Forum*, 28: 951–53.

Raphael, D, Steinmetz, B, Renwick, R, Rootman, I, Brown, I, Sehdev, H, Phillips, S and Smith, T (1999) The Community Quality of Life Project: a health promotion approach to understanding communities. *Health Promotion International*, 14 (3): 197–210.

Registered Nurses Association of Ontario (2002) *Establishing Therapeutic Relationships.* Ontario: RNAO.

Rogers, A, Bower, P and the EPP Evaluation Team (2006) *The National Evaluation of the Pilot Phase of the Expert Patients Programme: Final Report.* Manchester: NPCRDC.

Rogers, C R (1967) *On Becoming a Person. A Therapist's View of Psychotherapy.* London: Constable.

Roper, N, Logan, W W and Tierney, A J (2000) *Roper–Logan–Tierney Model of Nursing: The Activities of Daily Living Model.* Edinburgh: Churchill Livingstone.

Rowlands, G (2009) Health Literacy and Long-Term Conditions. *Primary Health Care,* 19 (7): 16–20.

Royal College of General Practitioners (2008) *Prognostic Indicator Guidance* [online]. Available at: www.goldstandardsframework.nhs.uk/Resources/Gold%20Standards%20Framework/PrognosticIndicatorGuidancePaper.pdf.

Royal College of Nursing (2003) *Defining nursing: def... Nursing is...* London: Royal College of Nursing.

Royal College of Nursing (2006) *Meeting the Needs of People with Learning Disabilities: Guidance for Staff.* London: Royal College of Nursing.

Salovey, P and Mayer, J D (1990) *Emotional Intelligence* [online]. Available from: www.unh.edu/emotional_intelligence/EIAssets/EmotionalIntelligenceProper?EI1990%20Emotional%20Intelligence.pdf [accessed: 2 August 2010].

Scherder, E and Van Manen, F (2005) Pain in Alzheimer's disease: nursing assistants' and patients' evaluations. *Journal of Advanced Nursing,* 52 (2): 151–58.

Scottish Government (2008) *Living and Dying Well: a National Action Plan for Palliative and End of Life Care in Scotland.* Edinburgh: The Scottish Government.

Scottish Government Health Delivery Directorate Improvement Support Team (2009) *Long Term Conditions Collaborative: High Impact Changes.* Edinburgh: The Scottish Government.

Scottish Intercollegiate Guidelines Network (2000) *Management of Early Rheumatoid Arthritis: A National Clinical Guideline.* Edinburgh: SIGN.

Scottish Intercollegiate Guidelines Network (2007) *Heart Disease Guidelines.* Edinburgh: SIGN.

Scottish Intercollegiate Guidelines Network (2009) *British Guidelines on the Management of Asthma.* Edinburgh: SIGN.

Simon, C, Everitt, H, Birtwhistle, J and Stevenson, B (2002) *Oxford Handbook of General Practice.* Oxford: Oxford University Press.

Smith, M K (1997, 2002) Paulo Freire and informal education. *The Encyclopaedia of Informal Education* [online]. Available from www.infed.org/thinkers/et-freir.htm [accessed: 18 October 2010].

Smith, P (1992) *The Emotional Labour of Nursing: How Nurses Care.* Worcester: The Macmillan Press Ltd.

Social Care Institute for Excellence and National Institute for Health and Clinical Excellence (2007) *A NICE-SCIE Guideline on Supporting People with Dementia and their Carers in Health and Social Care.* London: The British Psychological Society and Gaskell.

Sutherland, D and Hayter, M (2009) Structured review: evaluating the effectiveness of nurse case managers in improving health outcomes for three major chronic diseases. *Journal of Clinical Nursing,* 18 (21): 2978–92.

Telford, K, Kralik, D and Koch, T (2005) Acceptance and denial: implications for people adapting to chronic illness: a literature review. *Journal of Advanced Nursing,* 55 (4): 457–64.

Tennant, R, Hiller, L, Fishwick, R, Platt, S, Joseph, S, Weich, S, Parkinson, J, Secker, J and Stewart-Brown, S (2007) The Warwick–Edinburgh Mental Well-being Scale (WEMWBS): development and UK validation. *Health and Quality of Life Outcomes*, 5 (63).

Thomas, K (2003) *Caring for the Dying at Home: Companions on the Journey.* Abingdon: Radcliffe Medical Press.

Toofany, S (2006) Patient empowerment: myth or reality? *Nursing Management*, 13 (6): 18–22.

Turnock, A C, Walters, E H, Walters, J A and Wood-Baker, R (2005) Action plans for chronic obstructive pulmonary disease. *Cochrane Database Systematic Review*, 4: CD005074.

Valenti, L, Lim, L, Heller, R F and Knapp, J (1996) An improved questionnaire for assessing quality of life after myocardial infarction. *Quality of Life Research*, 11: 535–43.

Walker, A (ed.) (2005) *Understanding Quality of Life in Old Age.* Maidenhead: Open University Press.

Wallace, P (2001) Improving palliative care through effective communication. *International Journal of Palliative Nursing*, 7 (2): 86–90.

Watson, M, Haviland, JS, Greer, S, Davidson J and Bliss, M (1999) Influence of psychological response on survival in breast cancer: population based cohort study. *The Lancet*, 354: 1331–36.

Welsh Assembly Government (2003) *A Strategic Direction for Palliative Care Services in Wales.* Cardiff: Welsh Assembly Government.

Wilmot, J (2002) Palliative care of non-malignant conditions. In: Charlton, R (2002) *Primary Palliative Care: Dying, Death and Bereavement in the Community.* Abingdon: Radcliffe Medical Press.

World Health Organisation (2002) *National Cancer Control Programmes: Policies and Managerial Guidelines.* Geneva: World Health Organisation.

World Health Organisation (2009) *Milestones in Health Promotion: Statements from Global Conferences.* Geneva: World Health Organisation.

World Health Organisation (2010) *The Determinants of Health* [online]. Available from: www.who.int/hia/evidence/doh/en/ [accessed: 7 October 2010].

Yura, H and Walsh, M B (1973) *The Nursing Process: Assessing, Planning, Implementing, Evaluating.* New York: Appleton Century Crofts.

Index

Note: Page number in italics refers to figures, illustrations, and tables.